A MONOGRAPH

OF

DISEASES OF THE NOSE AND THROAT

BY

GEORGE H. QUAY, M. D.

Professor of Rhinology and Laryngology in The Cleveland Medical College; Member of the American Institute of Homœopathy, Ohio State Homœopathic Medical Society, Etc.

INDIAN EDITION

B. Jain Publishers Pvt. Ltd.
Delhi

Price : Rs. 35.00

Reprint Edition 2000

Published by :

B. Jain Publishers (P) Ltd.

1921, Street No. 10, Chuna Mandi,
Paharganj, New Delhi - 110055 (INDIA)
Ph. No. : 7770430, 7770572, 7536418

Printed in India by :
J.J. Offset Printers
Delhi

ISBN 81-7021-676-1

BOOK CODE B-2430

To

The Memory

of

Professor Nathaniel Schneider, M. D.,

My Preceptor and Early Guide

in the Study of Medicine

This Volume is Lovingly Dedicated

by The Author.

PREFACE

It has been the author's aim in the succeeding pages to present in concise form a Monograph on the Diseases of the Nose and Throat especially adapted to the needs of the student and the general practitioner.

The book is the outcome of an experience in the general practice of medicine which was not small, supplemented by several years of exclusively nose, throat and ear work. During the last five years I have been in almost daily contact with students, in the capacity of teacher, and have especially felt the need of a condensed work on the subject dealt with.

Few general practitioners have either the time or the inclination to wade through a volume on rhinology and laryngology which deals with exhaustive details, though a working knowledge of the diseases of the nose and throat is absolutely essential to the successful physician. I have, therefore, kept constantly in mind these two classes of readers.

Only enough anatomy and physiology is given to enable the reader to comprehend the text.

I have especially endeavored to emphasize throughout the work the necessity of treating the patient in his totality. It has, however, been my aim to impress on the reader the fact, that many diseased conditions met with in the nose and throat demand for their relief approved surgical treatment in addition to internal medication. Neither local nor general measures should, in my opinion, be used to the exclusion of the other.

To only a limited extent do I lay claim to originality.

In a monograph frequent reference to the authors consulted is impossible. I have freely availed myself of many of the works printed in the English language on diseases of the nose and throat, and of the journals devoted to this subject.

GEORGE H. QUAY

Cleveland, O.

PREFACE TO INDIAN EDITION

We are sure the reprint in India of this Monograph on the Diseases of the Nose & Throat, which was long out of market, will remove a long-felt want of a book which presents to its reader all the information he needs on the nose and throat. The author confined his practice exclusively to these human organs and is well qualified to write on the subject. We trust this book will prove of immense service to the students and practitioners.

PUBLISHERS

CONTENTS

CHAPTER XVI

CHAPTER XVII

CHAPTER XVIII

CHAPTER XIX

CHAPTER XX

LIST OF ILLUSTRATIONS

Chapter I

ANATOMY AND PHYSIOLOGY

The upper respiratory tract is composed of the anterior and posterior nasal fossæ, pharynx and the larynx.

The nose, the most prominent organ on the face, and the seat of the sense of smell, is formed of bone and cartilage, covered externally by muscles. It is divided by a cartilaginous and bony septum into two anterior fossæ.

The bones entering into the formation of the nose are, the two nasal, vomer, ethmoid, nasal process of superior maxillary and palate.

The cartilages are, two upper, two lower lateral, and the septal cartilage. Through the action of muscles upon these cartilages the openings of the nose can be dilated or contracted.

Extending into each fossa from the outer walls are three spongy bones called superior, middle and lower turbinals. The space between the lower turbinal and the floor of the nose is the lower meatus, between the middle and the lower turbinals the middle meatus, and between the superior and middle turbinals the superior meatus. Each fossæ has opening into it four sinuses, above the frontal, behind the sphenoidal, laterally the ethmoidal, and the maxillary or Antrum of Highmore.

The lachrymal duct extends from near the inner canthus of the lower eyelid to beneath the lower turbinal.

The mucous membrane lining the anterior nasal fossæ and cavities is called the pituitary membrane, from the nature of its secretions, or Schneiderian, from Schneider, the anatomist, who first demonstrated that the secretion came from the mucous membrane and not, as was supposed, from the brain.

The arteries are the anterior and posterior ethmoidal from the ophthalmic; they supply the frontal and ethmoidal sinuses and the roof of the nose; the sphenopalatine, from the internal maxillary, which supplies the mucous membrane covering the turbinals, the meatuses and the septum; the anterior septal, a branch of the superior coronary; and the alveolar branch of the internal maxillary which supplies the lining membrane of the antrum.

The veins, in the main, accompany the arteries.

The nerves are, the olfactory, which is the special nerve of the sense of smell, and is distributed over the upper third of the septum, and the superior, and upper part of the middle turbinals; and the nasal branch of the ophthalmic, which goes to the upper and anterior part of the septum. In addition, filaments from the anterior branch of the superior maxillary supply the lower turbinals and inferior meatuses; and the vidian supplies the upper and back part of the septum and the superior turbinals; the naso-palatine supplies the middle surface of the septum; the anterior palatine supplies the middle and lower turbinals.

The posterior nasal cavity or naso-pharynx, is the space extending from the posterior end of the anterior nasal cavities upward to the vault of the pharynx and downward to the free border of the soft palate forming three perpendicular walls, namely, the posterior and two lateral. Its mucous membrane is continuous with the anterior nares, but is much more abundantly supplied with glands than are the mucous membranes of the latter, which are called conglomerate and follicular. The former are situated near the orifices of the eustachian tubes; the follicular are on the posterior wall and vault of the pharynx. The eustachian tubes have their openings on the lateral walls of the pharynx on a line with the inferior meatus.

The isthmus of the fauces is the space between the lateral arches of the soft palate.

PHYSIOLOGY

The function of the anterior nasal fossæ is to warm and moisten the inhaled air, and by means of many little hairs, called vibrissæ, particles of dust and foreign bodies floating in the atmosphere are caught and thus prevented from entering the bronchial tubes and lungs. The particles which escape the vibrissæ are apt to be caught in the secretions and propelled outward by the peculiar action of the ciliated epithelium. This causes the desire to blow the nose, when they are expelled.

The nasal cavities are essential to the proper production of the voice. Clearness of voice depends almost wholly on the condition of these cavities. A swollen condition of the mucous membrane covering the turbinals, polypi, or a deflected or changed septum, produces the so-called "nasal-twang." Free nasal space is necessary as an aid to the sense of hearing. An occluded nostril prevents the proper rarefication of the air. The eustachian tube is simply a canal through which the air passes to the middle ear.

The nostrils are the seat of the sense of smell. The various parts of the nostrils supplied by the olfactory nerve are covered normally with a healthy secretion. The odoriferous particles coming in contact with this are dissolved, and thus brought in contact with the nerve terminals.

There are many ingenious theories offered to account for the sense of smell, but the above is the most generally accepted.

The oro-pharynx, or fauces, is that part of the respiratory and alimentary canal, which extends from the free border of the soft palate, to the fifth cervical vertebra behind, and the cricoid cartilage in front. Opening into it from above is the nasopharynx; in front the mouth; below the larynx and œsophagus.

Its arteries are derived from the external carotid.

The Palate. The roof of the mouth is composed of the hard and soft palates; the hard palate in front, is formed by the palatal process of the superior maxillary and palate bones. The soft palate is a muscular curtain covered by mucous membrane, attached to the hard palate. Hanging from the center of the posterior margin of the soft palate is a conical shaped muscular body called the uvula.

Arching outward and downward on each side from the site of the uvula, are two folds or curtains, called the anterior and posterior pillars.

The Tonsils. The faucial tonsils are two glandular bodies, one on each side, between the anterior and posterior pillars. Each has from five to fifteen crypts or openings on its faucial surface. The function of the tonsils is a mooted question.

The lingual tonsil is situated on the posterior surface of the base of the tongue, in front of and just above the superior free border of the epiglottis.

The pharyngeal, or sometimes called Luschka's tonsil, is located on the vault of the pharynx. When hypertrophied it frequently extends down the posterior and lateral walls.

The Larynx. The epiglottis is a turban shaped cartilaginous body covered with mucous membrane, and is attached below the base of the tongue by three muscles, two lateral and one central. The space between these muscular attachments to the epiglottis is called *valleculæ.* The upper free border of the epiglottis presents a variety of shapes, from almost horizontal, to the form of a letter W inverted. Extending posteriorly from the lower lateral free borders of the epiglottis are two folds called the ary-epiglottic folds; these terminate in two cartilages on each side, the anterior named the cartilage of Wrisberg and the posterior the cartilage of Santorini. Posteriorly between these cartilages is the interarytenoid fold. In this space will occasionally be found a small ulcer which will cause a persistent hacking cough.

The ventricular bands, or false cords, one on each side, extend antero-posteriorly, to the inner side and below the ary-epiglottic folds.

The vocal cords are two white or pearl-colored bands below the false bands, extending antero-posteriorly.

The ventricles of Morgagni are the two lateral depressions between the false bands and vocal cords.

Chapter II

METHOD OF EXAMINATION

Rhinoscopy is the art of examining the anterior and posterior nasal cavities.

Laryngoscopy is the art of examining the throat.

For proper examination of the nose and throat certain instruments are necessary. The first is, a good light. In this country the majority of rhinologists use electric light, gas or oil. For the purpose of concentrating the light a Mackenzie condenser (Fig. I), or some modification of it is needed. This can be used on an oil lamp with an Argand burner.

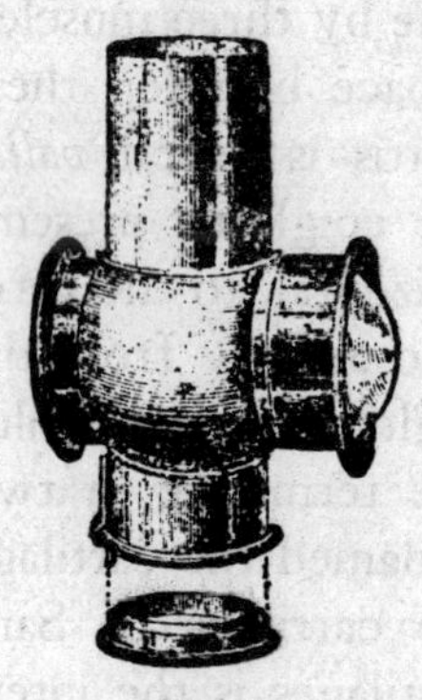

Fig. I

The second is, a three and one-half inch in diameter mirror. This is attached to a silk or rubber band worn around the head, the mirror to be adjusted so that the perforation in the center comes over the examiner's eye. Next the light is so to be placed that the condenser will be on the side of the patient and about on a plane with his eye. In place of the head band, the mirror may be attached to the end of an arm which has an enlargement made so as to fit over the upright metal part of the condenser.

In addition, a nasal speculum (of which there are a number of wire ones that usually answer the purpose) (Fig. II), aluminium probes or applicators (Fig. III), with roughened surface near the end for, retaining the cotton; and a tongue depressor are essential.

The Author's Tongue Depressor. (Fig. IV).

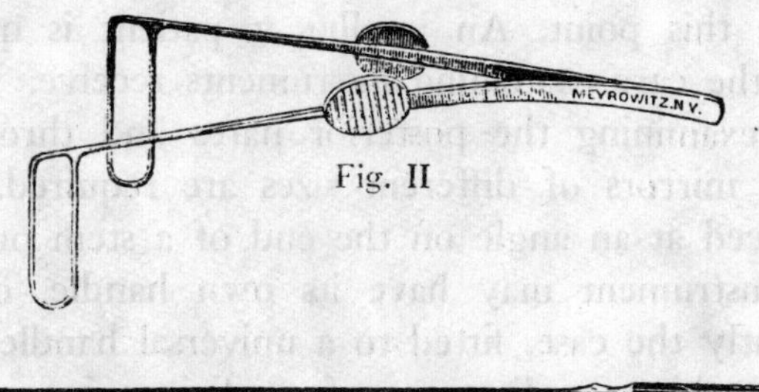

Fig. II

Fig. III

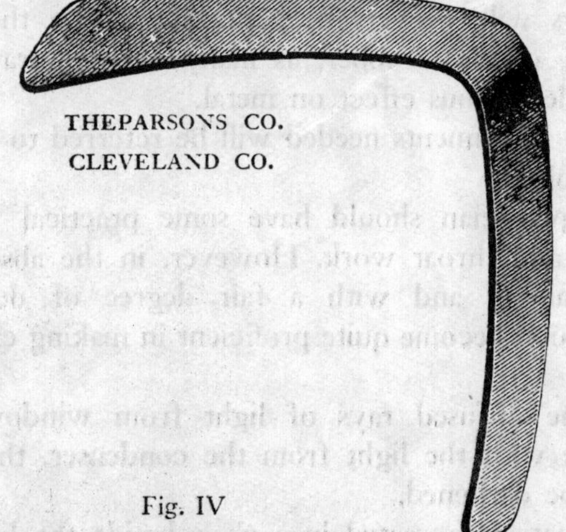

THEPARSONS CO.
CLEVELAND CO.

Fig. IV

The physician should be scrupulously clean with his instruments. After making an examination, thoroughly wash, and wipe clean, all instruments. I generally use a three to five per cent solution of Carbolic acid, for this purpose; the instrument is then wiped clean, held over the gas light, dipped into a separate glass containing a similar solution and finally wiped dry, when it is ready for the next patient. Too much stress cannot be laid on this point. An intelligent patient is quick to notice the care examining instruments receive.

For examining the posterior nares and throat four or five mirrors of different sizes are required. These are placed at an angle on the end of a stem or shank. Each instrument may have its own handle, or as is frequently the case, fitted to a universal handle.

For making applications of medicines in spray, an air receiver, pump, tubing and spray tubes are convenient. In their absence a half dozen hard rubber atomizers will answer. It is necessary that the tubes be made of hard rubber, as many of the sprays used have a deleterious effect on metal.

Other instruments needed will be referred to in their proper place.

The physician should have some practical training in nose and throat work. However, in the absence of such training and with a fair degree of dexterity, he can soon become quite proficient in making examinations.

As the diffused rays of light from windows will interfere with the light from the condenser, the room should be darkened.

The patient is seated in a chair beside the light, his knees placed together, with the examiner directly in front. Or the physician may separate his knees so that one will be on each side of the patient's knees; this is an inelegant position, but it allows the physician to get closer to the patient. I always lay a clean towel across my lap.

In examining the nose the first point to be noted is its shape. If the nasal bones have been fractured there will generally be some flattening or sinking in of the bridge, or possibly scars on the skin, which are the result of the injury responsible for the fracture. When the nose is crooked or pressed to one side there will be a deflection of the septum. The tip of the nose turned up, the so-called pugnose, is apt to be associated with atrophic rhinitis.

On examining the interior the examiner should note the color of the mucous membrane; and the shape of the septum (whether deflected or not); spurs, ridges or tumors on its surface should also be noted. Near its anterior extremity there is frequently a dry scab which the patient is apt to pick to relieve the feeling of itching. The ulcer caused by the removal of these scabs is a frequent cause of epistaxis.

The condition of the lower and middle turbinals is to be noted, *i.e.*, whether greatly swollen or in contact with the septum. Swollen or enlarged lower turbinals will prevent a view farther back. A thin pledget or layer of cotton, or what is better, a strip of lintine one and a half inches long by about one-half to one inch in width, which is saturated with a four per cent. Cocaine solution, and carried into the nostril and placed in contact with the enlargement. After about five minutes this pledget is removed, when the swelling will be found so reduced that a god view can be had of the middle turbinal. The physician is to notice if the latter is in contact with the septum. Frequently by tipping the patient's head slightly backward the upper turbinal can be seen.

In examining the mouth and posterior nares, notice the contour of the hard and soft palate. In case of a high arched palate there is usually a deflected septum. Where there is a bony ridge projecting down from the union of the palate bones, there is usually a ridge on the septum near the floor of the nostrils.

Next, the anterior pillars are to be inspected. When the pillars on each side are of a dusky red, or mottled colour, it is strongly suspicious of syphilis. The tonsils, when normal, should extend a little toward the median line from the pillars; if enlarged there may be an exudation at the mouth of the crypts. In chronic hypertrophy of the tonsils the anterior pillar is usually attached to the tonsil. On the posterior wall the colour of the mucous membrane is to be noted as well as the character of the secretion. In anæmic patients the cervical vertebræ are invariably prominent. Experience enables the examiner to observe all these points at a glance.

To examine the posterior nares the tongue is to be depressed, being careful not to carry the spatula too far back on the tongue. Unless this precaution is observed, the patient will gag, or he will elevate the border of the soft palate. A small or medium sized mirror, is warmed by hoding its reflecting surface over the flame, so as to prevent the condensation of moisture by the patient exhaling. It should never be carried into a patient's mouth until the physician first tests it on his own hand, or cheek. After properly heating the mirror is passed (reflecting surface upward) though the mouth. It is carried to one side of the uvula, being careful not to touch the palate. If the patient shows a tendency to retract the palate, he is to be requested to endeavor to breathe through the nose. A view of the posterior nares cannot always be obtained by one trial and it is often necessary to make several attempts. In fact, persons are sometimes met with where it is impossible to examine the posterior nares. After the mirror is properly placed the first object to appear is usually the posterior end of the septum; this should be narrow and somewhat wedge-shaped. By quickly changing the angle of the mirror the posterior extremities of the turbinals are seen. In hypertrophic conditions these are always enlarged. By raising the handle and depressing the mirror the vault of the pharynx can be seen. In the adult there may be bands and cords of cicatrical tissue, the remains of adenoid growths.

To examine the larynx the physician holds the patient's protruding tongue well forward by means of a napkin or towel, being careful not to press the frænum too strongly on the lower incisor teeth. One of the larger sized mirrors, with its reflecting surface downward, is then passed through the mouth until the back of the mirror elevates and presses backward the uvula. The handle of the mirror is to be carried to the left angle of the patient's mouth. This prevents the operator's hand from obscuring his line of vision.

The first image to be seen is that of the glands on the base of the tongue; then follows the epiglottis. The patient should now be requested to say, ah, or ā, as this effort will serve to raise the epiglottis and bring the larynx into view, and at the same time cause the vocal cords to come together.

Chapter III

ACUTE CATARRHAL RHINITIS

Synonyms. Acute nasal catarrh. Coryza. Cold in the head. Snuffles.

Definition. By acute catarrhal rhinitis is meant an acute inflammation of the mucous membrane lining the nasal cavities, of a catarrhal character, which sometimes implicates the adjacent sinuses and which frequently extends to the larynx.

Etiology. Sudden changes in the temperature, especially to cold accompanied by high winds; cold damp weather, such as we are accustomed to have during the spring and late fall months; cold wet feet; sitting in a draught when overheated, or sudden chilling of the body. In summer the disease is frequently caused by dust. Sitting or working in hot, close and ill-ventilated rooms, especially when heated by a hard coal baseburner, is also a frequent causative factor. So, too, is indigestion, especially if accompanied by constipation and over-loaded bowels. The latter, especially in children, I believe to be a frequent aggravating cause of catarrhal troubles. The daily wetting the hair tends to catarrhal diseases. Measles, smallpox and secondary stage of syphilis are usually ushered in by acute catarrhal symptoms.

Infants and children rarely have their legs properly protected in cold weather; when permitted to play or crawl on the floor it must not be forgotten that the temperature of the floor is from two to four degrees lower than other parts of the room. On account of its delicate organism the child is more susceptible than the adult to atmospheric changes.

There is also strong evidence tending to prove the infectious character of acute catarrhs.

Symptoms. After the age of childhood, one is usually conscious of catching cold. Generally there is some chilliness, depression, difficulty in getting warm; itching in the nose; sneezing, soon followed by stuffiness in nostrils, with watery discharge; chills running up and down the back, aching, etc. This stage is quickly followed by fever, during which the mouth and throat are apt to be dry; headache, and if the frontal sinuses are implicated the pain is worse over the brows. In the course of from twenty-four to forty-eight hours the nostrils may become totally occluded; this causes the voice to have a peculiar dead sound, the so-called "nasal twang."

Frequently the eustachian tubes become implicated, which causes some degree of deafness and pain. In many cases, especially in children, acute otitis is followed by perforation of the drum-head; otorrhœa and resulting impairment of hearing is a sequel. In the mojority of cases the conjunctivæ are implicated.

During the first stage the nasal secretion is thin and watery, which may be either bland or excoriating; after three or four days the secretion becomes thicker and assumes a yellowish color and occasionally is slightly blood-streaked. During this period the brow pain is intensified and there is a sense of fulness or pressure over the bridge of the nose. In nearly all instances the sense of smell is partially or wholly blunted, but returns on the subsidence of the nasal swelling. In the case of women the attack may be aggravated by spurting or dribbling of urine when coughing or sneezing; when this conditoin exists I advise the use of a napkin, so as to prevent the urine from coming in contact with the thighs.

Prognosis. An acute attack can usually be relieved in from three to five days, providing the patient has not chronic or hypertrophic rhinitis; if such is the case the attack is usually prolonged, the time depending on the degree of the chronic trouble.

In the case of nursing infants and old people, it is necessary to guard the prognosis. In infants the nostrils are blocked so that they cannot nurse and breathe at the same time. As a result they soon become debilitated and almost before one is aware of it, catarrhal pneumonia develops. Old people have not the vitality to withstand a severe cold and with them, as with children, the tendency is towards lung implication.

Treatment, Preventive. In those susceptible to colds, much can be done to prevent their occurrence. A cold chest and neck sponge both before dressing in the morning is excellent when counter-indications do not exist. In the debilitated, however, or if the bath is followed by chilliness and a feeling of languor, it must be used with great circumspection, if at all.

The feet should be kept warm and dry; to accomplish this, cork soles are invaluable. Daily changing of the hose and shoes also assists in keeping the feet warm. The practice of over-bundling the neck is pernicious, as is also the wearing of overcoats or heavy jackets indoors. Sleeping rooms should be thoroughly ventilated night and day

It is well to remember that old and feeble people demand warmer clothing than the robust, but it is better to have it light in weight.

The sooner a case is seen after its onset, with proper treatment, the shorter will be its course.

The laity usually consider a cold in the head of slight importance and endeavor to break it up by means of hot mustard foot-bath, hot lemonades, and a sweat. In some cases this will relieve the symptoms, but too often the attack lays the foundation, or is the beginning, of more serious trouble. This is especially so if there is a pre-disposition to disease of the respiratory tract.

When possible, keep the patient in his room or house, where the temperature is uniform and the air not too dry; let the diet be light. If constipated, a thorough hot water rectal injection is advisable; even though the bowels may be regular, it is a good plan to flush the rectum. It is often surprising what hard masses of fæcal matter will be brought away by a rectal flush, with a consequent relief of the catarrhal condition.

Inhaling Alcohol, Ammonia, or Menthol crystals will frequently aid in reducing the nasal swelling. A spray composed of Menthol and Cocaine, ten grs. each, to Albolene one oz. applied to the nasal cavities three or four times, at intervals of from one to two hours, will usually cut short, or materially modify an attack if used during the period of watery discharge. On the other hand, if used when the discharge is thick, I believe it serves to prolong the attack. When the Cocaine is used it is unwise to inform the patient of the fact.

When frontal pain is severe, due to blocking of the sinuses, steaming the face, or inhaling the steam through the nostrils, will frequently give relief. If the proper apparatus is not at hand to carry out this treatment, marked benefit may be derived from flannels wrung from hot water and held against the lower part of the forehead. To obtain continuous heat, it is well to cover the flannel with a rubber bottle containing hot water. After using the steam or heat, the patient should not be exposed to the cold for from twelve to twenty-four hours.

When convenient, the Turkish bath in the beginning will frequently cut short an attack.

Therapeutics

Camphor. In the beginning, chilly, feels as if catching cold. This remedy should be given in two drop doses of the θ on a lump of sugar every fifteen minutes until patient becomes warm. It is rarely advisable to administer more than three or four doses, when some other remedy will be indicated.

Kali iod., cum. merc. iod. Since this combination has not been proved, our indications are wholly clinical, I believe it to be a remedy of great value. After the Camphor stage, it will quickly cut short an attack characterized by sneezing; free watery bland discharge from nose; eyes may be implicated; occasional short hacking cough. The remedy must be stopped as soon as improvement begins.

Nux vomica. Sneezing, accompanied with fluent coryza during the day; may be itching in postnares with tickling cough. Stopped up at night; heavy pain over frontal region on account of implication of frontal sinuses.

Gelsemium. Epidemics in spring and fall; chilliness, especially up and down the back; must keep near the fire; no thirst; sneezing; discharge usually bland; muscles feel sore; head feels large; languid, does not want to move; heavy torpid condition; takes cold easily; tendency to neuralgia of the fifth pair of nerves.

Aconite. Attack frequently due to sudden changes of temperature; chilliness followed by fever, headache and sneezing; nose blocked up; restless and thirsty; dry, hacking cough.

Arsenicum alb. Free, watery, acrid, burning discharge; frequent sneezing; nose feels stopped up, but still it runs; redness around edge of nostril due to excoriating discharge; roof of mouth itches and burns. Feels the cold easily and wants to keep near the fire; prostration; especially useful in malarious districts.

Arsenicum iod. Frequently called for during epidemics. Similar to Arsc. alb. with added asthma; alternate chills and heat; sneezing is usually more violent than under *Arsc. alb.* The main indications to bear in mind are the irritating excoriating discharge and asthmatic tendency.

Ammonium carb. Acrid, watery discharge; sneezing during the day; burning in the eyes. At night discharge stops and nose is blocked up; must breathe through the mouth; the nightly blocking up causes a dry cough.

Ammonium brom. Similar to *Amm. carb.* and in addition, where colds always extend to larynx, this remedy in 1x trituration will usually prevent the laryngeal complications.

Euphrasia. Fluent coryza, with marked suffusion of

the eyes; great dread of light; conjunctivitis; the discharge from the nose is bland, while that from the eyes is acrid; feels like sneezing all the time.

Iodine. Dry coryza, which becomes fluent in open air; discharge hot; nose becomes sore; sneezing.

Kali iod. Profuse, acrid, watery discharge; violent sneezing; conjunctivæ, palate and eustachian tubes may be involved; strongly indicated if maxillary cavities are implicated.

Mercurius. Sneezing; profuse fluent corrosive discharge, worse at night. Later stages discharge is greenish; worse when warm in bed at night, yet cannot bear the cold.

Pulsatilla. Frequent alternation of fluent and dry coryza; sneezes as soon as he gets near the hot stove or heat, especially in the evening; feels better in cold air; later stages discharge yellowish.

Sambucus. Snuffles of infants; cannot breathe through the nose; starting, jumping in sleep from inability to breathe. I prefer this remedy in the 1x dilution.

SIMPLE CHRONIC RHINITIS

Synonyms. Chronic coryza. Chronic nasal catarrh.

Definition. By simple chronic rhinitis is meant a non-specific inflammation of the soft tissues of the nostrils, without new organization, which is usually accompanied by a similar condition in the pharynx and larynx.

Etiology. The disease is generally the result of repeated acute attacks or an uncured severe acute case, especially if occurring in those of poor general nutrition with debilitated constitutions. Certain occupations seem to favor it, as shops and factories, where the air is loaded with dust. Sexual excitement is likewise a predisposing factor in both sexes. In women the condition is frequently aggravated during the menstrual period and during pregnancy. There is evidently a close sympathy existing between the genital organs and the nasal erectile tissue, or corpora cavernosa.

Symptoms. Frequently the patient presents many of the symptoms manifest during a simple acute catarrh, except that in the chronic form they are more continuous. During damp, cold or changeable weather all the existing symptoms are greatly aggravated; there is more or less difficulty in breathing through the nose because of the swelling; there may be frequent sneezing; an excessive discharge is blown from the nostrils or drops posteriorly; the discharge from the nose is usually of a watery character, but may be thick, light or yellowish and occasonally slightly bloody. Frequent hoarseness, due to chronic laryngitis, or reflex from swelling of lower turbinals, or mucous membrane on the floor of the nostrils, is often present. Frontal headache is a common occurrence, and deafness with tinnitus is also a frequent accompaniment.

Diagnosis. This form of rhinitis is to be distinguished from the hypertrophic. In simple chronic rhinitis, the anterior part of the lower turbinals can be pressed back with the probe; there is, too, a decided shrinkage of the tissues for a short time after the application of cocaine. In the hypertrophic form, neither the pressure of the probe nor the application of cocaine causes decided collapse of tissue. In many cases, however, the simple form gradually merges into the hypertrophic.

Prognosis. The disease is readily controlled by proper and timely treatment. If neglected it not infrequently develops into the hypertrophic form.

Treatment. In all forms of catarrhal disease, cleanliness is of the first importance; the mucous membrane must be kept clean. The method for accomplishing this consists in the use of the anterior and posterior douche and spray. The anterior douche can be snuffed up the nostrils from the hand or a teaspoon. Or, a very good instrument can be made from a soft rubber catheter five or six inches long; tie one end, make ten or twelve small perforations two inches back from the tied end and to the other end attach a rubber bulb.

The posterior nasal syringe has more charges laid to its door than in my opinion facts justify. It is condemned by many because of the fear that it may cause otitis from water entering the eustachian tubes. A careful operator, by keeping the tip in the median line and using but little force, only enough to discharge the solution through the nostrils, while the patient is cautioned against throwing the head sideways, will rarely, if ever, cause otitis. The patient should also be instructed not to blow the nose immediately after the douche is used.

In using anteriorly a spray attached to the air condenser, the pressure should never be over ten pounds, as too much force increases rather than relieves the swollen condition. In my personal practice I never use the air condenser spray anteriorly, as I believe that better results are obtained by douching, or by means of the posterior spray.

For cleansing the membranes, *Bi-carbonate of soda* and *salt* (one-quarter of a teaspoonful of each to a cupful of warm water), or *Carbolic acid* (five to ten drops to a cupful of water), are most useful agents. Another excellent preparation is what is known as "Seiler's Tablets." The use of "Listerine" is also beneficial. Frequently the homœopathic remedy, administered internally, conjoined with thorough cleanliness, is all sufficient, yet there are cases where it is well to use a medicated coarse spray posteriorly; for this purpose five to twenty drops of the remedy which is being used internally, may be added to the ounce of sterilized water.

For use in the nasal spray many formulæ have been published. Although the careful prescriber may not have to use them, in the majority of instances their use is empirical, I have deemed it best to give a few of the local applications that have received recognition.

℞.	Ex. Pinus Canadensis,	gtt. xxx.
	Glycerine,	ʒii.
	Water,	℥i.
M.		
℞.	Sulphate zinc.,	gr. i.
	Water,	℥i.
M.		
℞.	Boric acid,	gr. x.
	Water,	℥i.
M.		
℞.	Hydrastis muriate,	gr. i.
	Water,	℥i.

M.

℞. Menthol crystals, gr. v. to xv.
Albolene, ℥i.

M.

℞. Terebene, gtt. x.
Albolene, ℥i.

M.

The numerous powders, so frequently recommended, I do not use, as I obtain better results from the spray.

If the turbinal swelling does not show a decrease within three or four weeks, it will be advisable to cocainize and make one or two incisions with the galvano-cautery point along the most prominent part of the lower turbinals. In doing this care must be exercised not to cauterize too broad a surface.

Dietetic and hygienic treatment must be observed; this point cannot be too strongly impressed upon the reader. Many of the victims of this form of disease are dyspeptics. The diet should be plain and nutritious, all highly seasoned articles being avoided. If fermentation of the stomach or bowels exist it should be corrected by a proper diet and the indicated remedy. Above all, constipation or sluggishness of the bowels must not be permitted.

Much can be done by the proper selection of the internal remedy. In its selection the prescriber should constantly keep in mind both the constitutional symptoms and the local lesions.

Therapeutics

Ammonium mur. Clear watery mucus running from

the nose, corroding the lips; loss of smell; left nostril swollen and sensitive to touch. Constant itching in the nose with desire to blow. Hoarseness, with burning in larynx.

Antimonium crud. Eczema, cracks around the nostrils; nose painful when breathing, as from inhalation of cold air or acrid vapors.

Antimonium sulf. aurat. Pimples or acne on nose. Nasal catarrh complicated with catarrh in the bronchial tubes.

Argentum nit. Sickly looking; chilliness; sneezing; headache; great itching in nose; discharge yellow, may be bloody.

Arsenicum iod. Predisposition to catch cold easily; ulceration inside of nose; burning, acrid discharge; asthma.

Calcarea carb. Offensive smell in nose, like rotten eggs; nose dry and obstructed at night, free during day. Discharge thick, fetid; cervical lymphatic glands enlarged. Scrofulous diathesis.

Causticum. Dry catarrh with obstruction of both nostrils, or fluent coryza with laryngo-tracheitis.

Ferrum met. Bleeding in morning on stooping; yellow face; face flushes easily. Lips pale. Anæmic patients.

Hamamelis. Varicose condition of blood vessels in nose and throat. Epistaxis with tightness in bridge of the nose.

Hepar sulph. Extremely susceptible to catarrhal attacks; sensitive to cold, open air or draughts. Much mucus, apt to be bloody.

Hydrastis Can. Discharge sticky, thick yellow. Tickling like a hair in the right nostril; sneezing, fulness over eyes, dull frontal headache; air feels cold in the nose.

Kali bich. Small ulcers on the septum; pain in root of the nose with obstruction. Ropy, tough discharge. When discharge is fluent excoriates the nose and lip. Sneezing in the morning on going into the open air. (A drug often prescribed when not indicated.)

Kali iod. When adjacent sinuses are involved, especially if nasal discharge stops and is followed by pain in sinuses; throbbing pain in nasal bones. Continuous watery discharge, usually acrid; sneezing; eustachian tubes may be involved; nocturnal aggravation; alternating heat and chilliness.

Mercurius bin. Discharge whitish-yellow or greenish, may be fetid and corrosive; nostril swollen. May have some degree of deafness; enlarged tonsils. Usually worse at night when warm, and in damp rainy weather.

Natrum arsen. Supra-orbital headache, eyes implicated, with a burning, watery discharge. Sensation constantly of nose stopped up; pain in the root of the nose.

Natrum carb. Thick yellow discharge; stoppage worse at night with sneezing. Worse from least draught of air; also on alternate days. Eruption on nose, around mouth and lips; red nose with white pimple, painful when touched.

Natrum mur. Absence of smell and taste. Hydroa around mouth or lips. Takes cold in head easily, with stoppage of the nose; very sensitive to either cold or warmth. Emaciated, great prostration, easily fatigued.

Phosphorus. Discharge green or bloody; sensation of fulness high up in left nostril; sneezing causes pain in the throat. Nose red, swollen. Hoarseness.

Pulsatilla. Thick yellow or yellowish-green discharge, usually bland; discharge has bad smell. During the evening or in a warm room stoppage of nostrils occurs, but the thick discharge is increased in the morning.

Rhus tox. In the rheumatic subject every change of the weather aggravates the catarrhal trouble; sneezing worse at night; may be fever blisters or crusts under the nose. Puffiness of nose.

Sanguinaria nit. Coryza with pain in root of the nose and frontal sinuses; sneezing; burning in nostrils; whitish, raised patches on the mucous membrane of the nostrils and roof of the mouth. Laryngitis; dry, tickling cough; loss of voice.

Selenium. Itching in nose and edges of nostrils; complete obstruction of nose, finally ending in diarrhœa.

Sepia. Very sensitive to odors; nose-bleed during menses or pregnancy. Fluent coryza with sneezing in early morning.

Sticta Pulmon. Fulness in nose with dry mucous membrane; constant desire to blow the nose, but no discharge results. Dry cough at night.

Sulphur. Fluent discharge, sneezing, nostrils burn and itch, watery discharge outdoors; stopped up indoors; feels suffocated in the house. Catarrhal symptoms get better, then worse.

Theridion. Offensive yellowish or yellowish-green discharge. Watery discharge with sneezing in evening.

HYPERTROPHIC RHINITIS

Definition. The term hypertrophic rhinitis signifies a

chronic inflammation of the tissues lining the nasal cavities, characterized by structural changes.

Etiology. The changes which characterize the disease usually result from long-continued chronic rhinitis, though all cases of chronic rhinitis do not terminate in the hypertrophic form. The use of snuffs, especially those containing mineral astringents; and local lesions, as deflected septum, spurs or ridges of the septum, etc., must also be noted as causative factors.

Pathology. Organization takes place in the thickened tissues and new blood vessels are formed. Even the periosteum is thickened. The hypertrophied condition is not uniform, and is usually more pronounced on the free borders of the middle and lower turbinals. These changes do not take place suddenly, and often require years.

Symptoms. The most prominent symptom is difficult nasal breathing. This is due to the hypertrophy of the tissues and to the thick tenacious secretion; frequently the nostrils become so occluded that the patient can neither inhale nor exhale through the nose. This closing of the nostrils is especially noticeable when lying down. The blocking of the nose causes so-called "mouth breathing," with resulting dry, coated tongue. The sense of smell is diminished or wholly lost, and the sense of taste is frequently impaired. Periodical frontal headache of a neuralgic character is often marked; this is especially true in hypertrophy of the middle turbinals. Tinnitus is usually present, and nearly all cases are characterized by some degree of deafness. The posterior nares are generally implicated, with resulting dropping of mucus in the throat, which is worse in the morning soon after getting up, or after breakfast. The movements of the pharyngeal muscles, due to eating and swallowing, causes the mucus on their surfaces to become detached.

Ocular neuralgia, conjunctivitis and asthenopia are frequent; the eye symptoms, when due to this cause, will remain unrelieved until proper treatment is directed to the nose. Impaired memory and inability to fix the attention are often present. Hoarseness is common, and is due to implication of the larynx, or is reflex from varicoses of the posterior end of the lower turbinals. It may also be due to the lower turbinal coming in contact with the floor of the nose. Asthma is frequently present; in fact, many authorities claim that in over ninety per cent. of asthmatic cases the cause can be found in an abnormal condition of the anterior and posterior nares. In my own experience, a large majority of the cases of asthma met with have been decidedly relieved by treatment directed toward pathological conditions, of whatever character, in the nasal cavities.

Rhinoscopy. Anterior examination reveals enlarged lower turbinals. To obtain a view farther back it is necessary to reduce this enlargement, by placing in contact with it a strip of cotton saturated with a four per cent. *Cocaine* solution; after four or five minutes the cotton can be removed, when the middle turbinal will come into view, revealing its anterior end very much enlarged, probably firmly in contact with the septum, and not infrequently presenting much the appearance of a polypus with a broad attachment. In addition, polypi may be present in the hypertrophied area.

Posteriorly there is presented a mulberry-like enlargement of the posterior ends of the lower turbinals. These enlargements are due to a varicose condition of the tissues; when they impinge on the septum, the patient usually has paroxysms of sneezing. It should not be forgotten that if *Cocaine* has been used in the nostrils this posterior swelling may largely disappear. In many cases the middle turbinals partake of the appearance of the lower turbinals, but not in so marked a degree.

The walls of the septum present a light colored swelling which gives them the appearance of large blisters. This, in connection with the enlarged turbinals, is a frequent cause of nasal stenosis.

Prognosis. Generally good, with aid of proper surgical treatment. By such treatment the patient can be given enlarged breathing space, deafness can be held in check and in many cases the hearing can be improved.

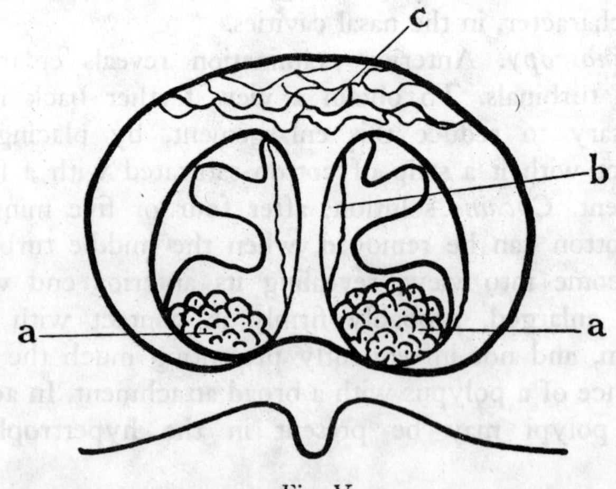

Fig. V

Treatment. In the main the treatment is surgical. The enlargement, whether soft tissue, cartilage or bone, must be removed. The patient's health will be compromised if in these conditions the physician adhere too tenaciously to the internal remedy, and exclude approved surgical treatment.

Before beginning an operation in the nasal cavities they should be sprayed or swabbed with *Peroxide of Hydrogen* one part, to distilled water three parts, the resulting foam being wiped off with dry pledgets of cotton; then by means of "Lintine" or absorbent cotton flattened (in size somewhat larger than the area to be treated), a four to six per cent. cocaine solution is applied by the aid of a proper light to the surface to be treated, the dossil being allowed to remain in direct contact with the part for from five to eight minutes. It is well to have the patient incline his head slightly forward so as to prevent the cocaine from trickling down the pharynx. After the removal of the cotton and before cauterization, the membrane is to be dried with cotton. Spraying the nostrils with a cocaine solution should not be done, as by so doing there is greater liability of the solution entering the pharynx, which will cause a sense of constriction and an increased desire to clear the throat. Formerly I used twelve to twenty per cent. solutions of cocaine, but during the past few years I rarely find it necessary to use one stronger than eight per cent., generally four per cent., thus lessening the danger of systemic disturbance. I believe its anæsthetic effect to be as thorough as when the stronger solutions are used.

The methods used for removing the hypertrophies

are, galvano-cautery, acids, snare, various forms of knives, cutting forceps (Fig. VI) and scissors (Fig. VII). It is usually better to begin treatment in the anterior nares and work back. Before making caustic applications, albolene or some clean oil should be gently swabbed on the opposite surface, and unless the operator has a steady hand, a nasal speculum with a long blade to protect the opposite surface is quite necessary.

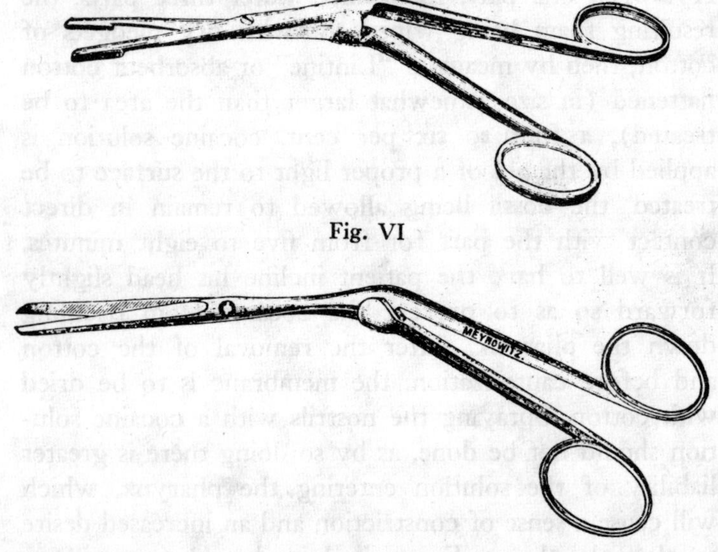

Fig. VI

Fig. VII

For the anterior hypertrophy on the lower turbinals, after proper cleansing and cocainizing, the platinum point heated by the galvano-cautery battery is preferable. Carrying the point as far back as desired for one sitting, the current is turned on and the knife brought forward to the end of the turbinal, making a deep incision; the current must not be turned off before the knife is taken from the tissues. When the battery is supplied with a proper rheostat to regulate the heat in the platinum point, which should be of a dull cherry-red color, the bleeding is trifling. For a few hours after the treatment, a loose pledget of cotton or lambs' wool should be lightly pressed into the nostril to prevent dust or foreign particles lodging on the cut surface. The succeeding treatments should be at least one week apart. Scabs must not be torn off, as by doing so the reparative process is prolonged. For enlargements of the anterior part of the middle turbinal, the cold wire snare may be used. As the wire is apt to slip off the mucous membrane, it is necessary to make a slight cut with the scissors through the tissue, one-half to one inch back from the end; this cut enables the wire loop to get a bite without slipping. By slowly turning the screw on the snare (consuming fully one hour in cutting through), the after bleeding will be slight.

The acids to be preferred are, chromic, tri-chloracetic and glacial acetic; the two former are never to be used on the septum, as their destructive action is so great they are liable to cause perforation.

For the acid treatment, the parts are to be prepared as for the galvano-cautery. I prefer to use the acids in solution; a few drops of water will liquefy an ounce of the crystals.

A small bit of cotton should be wound around the end of the applicator, so as to be not larger than a kernel of wheat. This is dipped in the acid and firmly pressed, for about ten seconds, on the surface to be reduced; in withdrawing the applicator from the nose care must be exercised not to cauterize the edge of the nostril. During the application of the acid the patient should breathe through the mouth, thus preventing the fumes from the acid from being drawn through the nostril which, if it occurs, is liable to increase the irritation and cause sneezing. It is rarely necessary to cover a broad space with the acid, but better to make a long, narrow cauterization. In from four to seven days the first scab will come off, the enlarged tissue on each side of the cavity left by the slough gradually contracting by the cicatrix, and appearing not unlike the gums around the cavity of an extracted tooth. When necessary to reapply the acid it should be brought in contact with the part first treated, as it is not advisable to destroy a large surface of the mucous membrane.

After acid applications there is usually, for a few hours, some pain in the nose, and it may extend to the cheek and forehead.

For posterior hypertrophies (Fig. V, *a.*), the cold wire snare is the best instrument (Fig. VIII). The loop is carried through the anterior nares, and by the aid of the rhinoscope, or by the sense of touch, is made

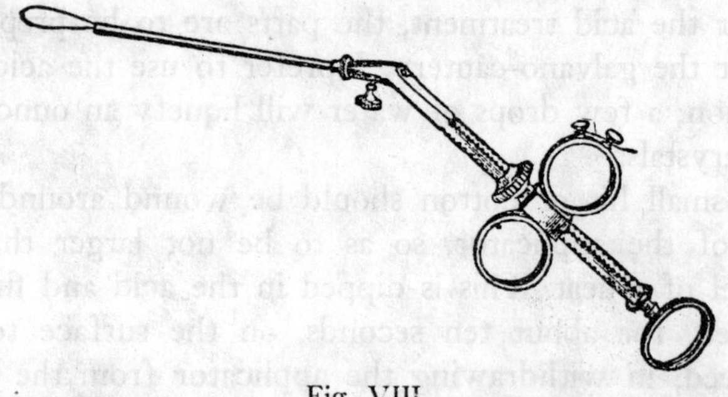

Fig. VIII

to encircle the hypertrophy. Occasionally the operator can pass his index finger through the patient's mouth and direct the loop around the varix. Simple as it appears, it is frequently a very difficult matter to snare the hypertrophy. When the loop is in place, at least an hour should be consumed in dividing the mass; by this slow process hemorrhage is entirely avoided. Acid applications to the posterior end of the lower turbinal must be made with the greatest care, in order that the acid may not approach too near the eustachian orifice, thus causing acute otitis. The swellings on the sides of the septum posteriorly (Fig. V, *b.*) are best treated with acetic acid on cotton wrapped applicator; if the patient can control his palate so that the posterior mirror can be used, they can be satisfactorily treated with the galvano-cautery.

All spurs or ridges on the septum coming in contact with the opposite wall are to be removed by the saw, scissors or trephine. If the operator has a motor the trephine is much more satisfactory than either the saw or scissors. The scissors or the knife to trim the inequalities left by the trephine is usually necessary.

As the nose is abundantly supplied with blood-vessels, bleeding is apt to be quite profuse after the cutting or the sawing operation. It can generally be controlled by using in the nose a spray of *Peroxide of Hydrogen*, or when this fails, by carrying well back into the nostrils a tampon of lambs' wool two to three inches long, and of a thickness to snugly fit in the nostril saturated with *Peroxide of Hydrogen.**

* For other means used in controlling nasal bleeding the reader is referred to the chapter on Epistaxis.

Tampons should not be allowed to remain in the nose longer than twenty-four hours; before being removed they must be softened with an antiseptic douche, so as to prevent the fibers of the wool from dislodging the eschar, which might cause secondary hemorrhage. Until the parts operated on are healed, an antiseptic douche should be gently used every morning and evening.

When deafness is present, the medicated air blast, or the Politizer bag, should be resorted to every second or third day for the purpose of opening the eustachian tubes; if the use of the air blast or the Politizer bag fails to open them and space through the nostrils permit, the eustachian catheter should be used.

General Treatment and Therapeutics. All that has been said under the head of Chronic Rhinitis applies equally well to the hypertrophic form.

ATROPHIC RHINITIS

Synonyms. Atrophic catarrh. Dry catarrh. Fetid catarrh.

Definition. The term atrophic rhinitis signifies an atrophy or washing away, more or less, of the mucous membrane, glands and turbinal bones of the nasal cavities, which is frequently accompanied by a diseased condition of the accessory sinuses, and the pharynx.

Etiology. Atrophic rhinitis is occasionally the result of the hypertrophic form. Other causes are: living or working in ill-ventilated rooms; working in the fumes of tobacco; smoking, alcoholism and syphilis. When due to the latter cause it is frequently accompanied by ozæna. Personally I believe that in the majority of cases occurring in children, there is an inherited syphilitic or a scrofulous taint. When it occurs in young girls puberty is generally delayed.

In many of these cases the tip of the nose is turned up, the so-called pug-nose; this condition is not due to disease, but is congenital, the peculiar shape predisposing to the disease. I have seen numerous cases where the atrophic condition was due to the indiscriminate destruction of the mucous membrane by caustics, and to amputation of the lower and middle turbinals. When occurring prior to puberty a larger per cent. of cases are seen in girls than in boys.

Pathology. The peculiar feature is the dryness of the mucous membrane. This is due to atrophy or destruction of the glands and follicles, which are abundant in the nose; also to the non-development, or surgical destruction of the turbinal bones.

Symptoms. Anterior rhinoscopy reveals a dry, shriveled condition of the membranes. Frequently the cavities are so enlarged that the posterior pharyngeal wall can be seen through the nostrils. In many cases the anterior ends of the turbinals become almost completely absorbed. There is not the congestion and hypertrophy found in other forms of rhinitis. Instead, thin, dry crusts of mucus and scales are seen adhering to the nasal walls, which are difficult to remove. Usually the most annoying symptom to the patient is the excessive dryness of the nostrils. Nose-bleed is a frequent result of picking the septum to remove the crusts, or of the irritation due to dryness; often there is a partial or total loss of the sense of smell and taste, and not infrequently some degree of deafness is present. Depression of the system may result, due to absorption of the fetid secretion. When ozæna is present, the patient is usually not aware of the bad odor, unless his attention has been called to it. In perhaps the majority of cases the pharynx presents the same atrophic condition.

Prognosis. Of course much depends on the age of the patient, occupation and the duration of the atrophic condition, as well as on the thoroughness with which proper treatment is carried out. In cases of long standing, with decided atrophy, a cure is out of the question; but when the change is recent a decidedly favorable prognosis can be given. In those cases which cannot be cured much can be done to relieve the dryness and formation of scabs, and to prevent the fetid odor. Occasionally it becomes necessary in contending with the odor to persist in local treatment throughout life.

Treatment. The treatment is both local and systemic. In the local treatment of first importance is cleanliness. This cannot be too strongly insisted upon for, to obtain good results, it must be thorough. Crusts must be removed by the anterior, or the posterior nasal douche; it is frequently necessary to use both. One excellent solution for removing the hardened mucus is common salt, ten to twenty grains, borax five to ten grains, warm water four to six ounces. The preparation in the market known as "Listerine" is excellent. When ozæna is present, permanganate of potash five grains, to warm water one ounce, will usually prevent the fetor. When the above treatment fails to dislodge the crusts, hydrogen peroxide carried into the cavities on cotton will usually soften them so that they can be washed off. After they are thoroughly removed, the membranes should be dried with absorbent cotton wrapped on an applicator. When the nostrils are cleansed the indications are to use applications which will prevent the reformation of crusts, and also stimulate the dried membranes. For the former a pledget of absorbent cotton, or better still, lambs' wool, about the size of the little finger, is to be carried into the nostrils; this may be used dry or saturated with Glycozone or c.p. Glycerine, and allowed to remain in the nostrils from one-half to two hours. When the tendency is for the crusts to rapidly reform, the cotton pledget may be used once or twice a day for the first few weeks, after the cleansing douche; later every third or fourth day will answer. As a stmulating application, nitrate of silver, ten to forty grains, to water one ounce, can be applied to the mucous membrane by means of a swab once a day; frequently the stronger solution can be tolerated where the weaker causes pain. In many cases very good results can be had from local application, morning and night, of Ichythol ten to thirty drops to Albolene one ounce; or Bichloride of mercury one-half grain to Albolene one ounce. The Ichythol and mercury should be used with a vaporizer.

When crusts form on the cartilaginous septum, causing bleeding and ulceration, a cerate of yellow oxide of mercury ten grains, to fresh lard one ounce, or a calendula or hamamelis cerate, applied two or three times a day, will usually promote healing; but the patient must be enjoined not to pick or irritate the scab. As a base for cerates I prefer fresh lard to the commonly used vaseline. In refining the latter, sulphuric acid is used, and as this is not thoroughly eliminated, the vaseline preparations are apt to irritate the mucous membrane.

In all cases, hygiene and dietetics play an important part in the treatment. If anæmia, good nourishing food must be taken, and one of the cod liver oil preparations should be used at meal time.

When this disease occurs in adults they should be made to understand that the treatment may extend over a period of months, and occasionally, at varying intervals, for years.

Therapeutics

Alumina. Old people, hard, yellowish-green discharge, nose swollen and sore, septum ulcerated. In women catarrh and leucorrhœa alternate. Chronic constipation.

Argentum nitricum. Ulcers bleed when picked; loss of smell; locally to ulcers.

Aurum. Caries of nasal and palate bones due to syphilis; bones of face sore to pressure; nose blocked with discharge of blood; melancholia, low spirited; (muriate in scrofulous, ill-nourished). The prominent indications are, syphilitic diathesis, abuse of mercury and the melancholia.

Hepar sulph. Bones of nose sensitive to touch; after abuse of mercury; face apt to be of a dirty yellow color. Good remedy when mercury is indicated, but does not relieve.

Kali bich. Severe pain across the bridge of nose, discharge of plugs apt to be bloody, nasal membrane covered with little ulcers. Frequently indicated when the antrum is implicated.

Kali iodide. Secondary and tertiary syphilis; nose

swollen; tightness with throbbing in nasal bones; ulceration of septal cartilage; enlarged cervical glands. In this disease I have obtained the best results in the 1x or 2x trituration.

Mercury. Offensive odor; heavy pain in cheek bones and frontal sinuses; enlarged tonsils; torpid liver.

Nitric acid. Syphilitic ozæna, discharge very offensive; nose and throat dry; swelling in nose; bleeds on slightest touch; pale or yellow face after abuse of mercury.

Silicea. Great dryness of nose; apt to be stuffed, with loss of smell; scrofulous cases; nasal bones ulcerated; induration of glands. I prefer the 30x potency of this remedy.

As intercurrent remedies, *Calcarea carb.*, *Calcarea phos.*, *Ferrum*, *Sulphur*.

STRUMOUS RHINITIS OF CHILDREN

Synonyms. Sub-acute and chronic purulent rhinitis.

Definition. By strumous rhinitis of children is meant a sub-acute or a chronic inflammation of the nasal organs, characterized by a somewhat thick, yellowish, or greenish discharge, with a tendency to acute exacerbations.

Etiology. In the main, authorities are inclined to the opinion that the disease is disposed to manifest itself in children of an hereditary scrofulous, tuberculous, or syphilitic taint. Leucorrhœa in the mother will cause it. It is frequently developed during, or soon after, an attack of diphtheria, scarlet fever or measles.

Symptoms. During the early stage there are present

many of the symptoms which characterize acute rhinitis, but as the disease progresses the nasal discharge from both nostrils assumes a decidedly yellowish or purulent character, which excoriates the edges of the nostrils and the upper lip. During sleep the secretions become dry, thus blocking the nostrils and compelling the little patient to breathe through his mouth. In many of these cases there is associated with the rhinitis enlarged faucial and pharyngeal glands, and not infrequently the glands of the neck become implicated also; also, some degree of deafness is present in nearly all cases. On account of the absorption and swallowing of the mucus, plus the predisposing cause, the child is apt to have a pale and sickly appearance. When the age of puberty is reached, the condition, in perhaps the majority of instances, assumes an atrophic form.

A foreign body in the nose might be mistaken for strumous rhinitis, but in the former the discharge is usually from but one nostril, while in the latter both nostrils are involved.

Prognosis. If treatment is begun and followed during the early years of the disease the outcome is generally favorable, but if allowed to progress the tendency is towards atrophic rhinitis. When this condition is reached the prospect of a cure is less encouraging.

Treatment. The proper cleansing of the nostrils is an essential feature of the treatment, although this is often difficult to perform with children. To accomplish it any simple alkaline wash will answer, as boric acid, or salt, five grains of each to an ounce of boiled water. "Listerine" is also excellent. Sprays and atomizers in these cases are usually not advisable, as better results can be obtained by using a common rubber-bulb ear syringe, or a glass piston syringe having a blunt point. Of course the solution should be warm.

Frequently, as a means of cleansing the nostrils, the child can be made to sneeze, by using a pinch of snuff, or gently tickling the nose. In a tractable patient a bit of cotton wrapped on an applicator, and gently carried into the nostril with a rotary motion, will serve to dislodge the secretion.

General dietetic and hygienic measures should receive careful attention. Sweets and over-indulgence in any one kind of food must not be permitted; let the food be plain but nutritious. Due attention must be given to bathing and clothing; woollen under-garments should be worn during the summer and winter. As the victims are often poorly nourished it is usually advisable to keep them from school; they should be kept out-doors as much as possible. When convenient a change of air is often beneficial. At as early an age as possible the child should be taught to keep the nostrils clean by means of a handkerchief.

When the neck glands are enlarged and the abdomen is protuberant some preparation of cod liver oil will prove beneficial. When there are co-existing hypertrophy of the faucial tonsils, and adenoid vegetations in the vault of the pharynx, they must first be removed by amputation, and curettement.

Therapeutics

Arum triphyllum. Ichorous discharge, excoriating nose and lip; nose stopped up; discharge may be thick, yellowish, streaked with blood.

Bromium. Coryza, excoriating discharge, soreness on margins of the nose and upper lip. Acne on face. Scrofulous children with enlarged parotid and thyroid glands. Particularly indicated in scrofulous children, fair skin, light hair. Children subject to spasmodic or false croup.

Calcarea carb. Nose and upper lip swollen; clear, watery secretion, alternating with stoppage; or may be thick, purulent and fetid. Fat, scrofulous children, inclined to nose-bleed; history of delayed dentition, and sweaty occiput. Frequent diarrhœa, stools soft, whitish or yellowish-gray; or may be dry, hard and clay-like.

Calcarea hypophos. Anæmic, large head. open fontanels, dry, towy hair, abdomen distended; chronic diarrhœa, debility, lack of nervous energy. Strumous diathesis well marked.

Calcarea iod. Enlargement of lymphatic glands, nodular tonsillar hypertrophy, adenoid vegetations.

Calcarea phos. Tall, pale, anæmic children; nose swollen, nostrils sore; thick, yellowish-white mucus, pale, flabby, hypertrophy of tonsils; swelling of cervical and sub-maxillary glands; hoarseness.

Cina. Boring in the nose with the finger; even during sleep the child picks at the nose; grinding of the teeth and tossing about, and starting during sleep; cross, irritable, nervous excitement. I have frequently noticed relief by giving *Santoninum*, 4x trituration, three or four days, followed by *Cina*, 30x or higher, one dose every alternate day.

Bacillinum. During the past two years I have used this remedy in a few cases with apparently decided relief. My method is to give five or six pills of the CC once every eight days for five or six times, which is followed by one of the lime or mercurial preparations. The indication for the virus is the general tubercular appearance of the child; feverish at night; enlargement of the neck and abdominal glands; takes cold easily; perspiration at night on back or chest.

Kali iod. Mucus, watery or colorless, profuse, acrid, excoriating the nostrils and affecting the conjunctivæ; loss of smell; ozæna; marked periodicity. The 2x or 3x trituration, a two-grain powder twice a day.

Also consult the therapeutics given under Simple Chronic Rhinitis.

Chapter IV

EPISTAXIS

Synonyms. Rhinorrhagia. Nose-bleed.

Definition. Epistaxis signifies a bleeding or hemorrhage from the nose.

Etiology. Epistaxis is merely a symptom and may be due to a variety of causes. It may be traumatic, the result of operations within the nostrils, or direct force with or without fracture of the framework of the nose. It is also caused by fracture of the base of the skull, and may be the result of cerebral jar or concussion without direct violence of the nose.

Spurs or ridges of the septum, or deviation of the septum when in contact, or when strongly pressing on the opposite wall, may cause abrasion of the mucous membrane with resulting bleeding. Picking or removing scabs or hardened mucus from the septum is also a frequent cause.

Nasal bleeding is of frequent occurrence in passing from a dense to a rarefied atmosphere, as witnessed in ascending high altitudes.

In women epistaxis may take the form of vicarious menstruation, and may recur with the same periodicity as the normal discharge; or it may result from repelled skin eruptions and from astringent applications to bleeding piles.

In many cases of the acute diseases, as diphtheria, scarlet fever, typhoid fever, smallpox and pneumonia, epistaxis is often an early symptom. When occurring in the later stages of these diseases it indicates a serious condition.

Epistaxis may be symptomatic of valvular disease, or over-action of the heart; of congestion and other diseases of the liver and kidneys, and of degeneration of the coats of the blood vessels, especially in advanced life.

Malignant disease of the nose, and, occasionally, syphilitic rhinitis are accompanied by epistaxis. From personal observation, I believe, uncomplicated mucous polypi rarely causes epistaxis.

Symptoms. The bleeding may be quite slight, or so profuse as to cause fainting. This usually stops the hemorrhage. But, as stated by Bosworth, "It should be borne in mind, that, when syncope occurs, the blood may continue to flow into the air passage below, involving the danger of a new complication."

When the result of trauma, or due to local conditions, the bleeding usually occurs from one nostril. But when due to systemic conditions the bleeding may occur from both nostrils. Epistaxis frequently follows, and relieves, congestive headache.

Prognosis. When epistaxis is the result of an operation, or when due to trauma, it is easily controlled. But when it is met with as a symptom of the hemorrhagic diathesis, or occasioned by organic visceral lesions, the prognosis necessarily depends on the exciting cause. When occurring in advanced life, especially if there is associated visual disturbance, it usually presages cerebral hemorrhage. Vicarious epistaxis is usually relieved after the normal menstrual discharge is established. It must not be forgotten that the loss of large quantities of blood may so debilitate the system as to lay the foundation for, or aid in, developing more serious disease.

When epistaxis frequently recurs in young children a microscopic examination of the blood should be made to determine the presence or absence of hæmophilla.

Treatment. When called to treat a case of epistaxis it is necessary to ascertain the exciting cause, and if possible to locate the point from which the bleeding occurs. As vicarious epistaxis is an effort of nature to relieve the system, it should not be stopped unless the bleeding is alarming. Here the treatment should be directed to the underlying cause. The same rule should be followed when the bleeding is due to cerebral congestion. In moderately severe cases the patient should remain standing, or sitting with the head inclined slightly forward so as to prevent the blood entering the throat. If faintness occurs, of course the recumbent position (lying on the bleeding side) must be assumed. All clothing constricting the neck should be loosened. In the majority of cases, not due to operation, the bleeding point will be found on the lower part of the septal cartilage, about one-half to three-fourths of an inch from the nasal opening. When occurring from this place it can usually be relieved by firm pressure on the outside of the nose. Frequently it is advisable to first insert over the bleeding spot a tampon of iodoform gauze, lambs' wool or non-absorbent cotton, the cotton being smeared with calendula. When the bleeding is from the anterior septal artery, and continued firm pressure fails to stop it, the surrounding membrane will have to be cleansed, cocainized, and the bleeding point touched with chromic, trichlor-acetic or mono-chloracetic acid. Bleeding from the septal artery can frequently be stopped by firm pressure on the upper lip, first placing a pledget underneath the lip. As the superior coronary arteries anastomose, it is necessary that pressure be applied the whole length of the lip. Among the simple means that will prove sufficient in many cases of accidental or slight epistaxis, may be mentioned tannic acid, or burnt alum blown into the nostril; and ice or a cold key applied to the cervical region. Ice or cold water applied to the nose may also be of service. The patient standing erect with his arms perpendicular will frequently stop the bleeding. The introduction of cobwebs into the nostril, so generally used as a domestic remedy, will often arrest the hemorrhage. Freshly expressed lemon juice applied locally has been claimed to quickly arrest nose-bleed. Antipyrine, five per cent. solution, applied by means of an atomizer, has given relief. Nasal bleeding the result of operations in the nostrils is best controlled by tampons of antiseptic gauze or lambs' wool saturated with hydrogen peroxide, antipyrine or fluid extract of ergot. The tampon must be large enough to extend beyond, and make firm pressure on, the bleeding surface. The pledget may be allowed to remain twenty-four to forty-eight hours. The tampon loosely applied within the nostril will not answer the purpose. It is necessary that the pledget be firmly packed over the bleeding surface. Before removing the tampon it must first be thoroughly softened with an antiseptic or alkaline douche. As the fibres adhere to the cut surface, the plug must not be forcibly pulled out, but removed by a gentle rotary movement. To stop bleeding from post-operation wounds it is not advisable to use cocaine, as after its use secondary hemorrhage is likely to follow. The perchloride of iron should rarely, if ever, be used, as the blood soaks through it, thus causing a dirty mass which is disagreeable, and which may excite reflex irritation.

When the bleeding arises from the posterior portion of the nostril, and all other means fail to arrest it, tamponing the posterior nares may be resorted to. Bellocq's canula, so frequently described, but rarely used, is not necessary. As a substitute, a soft rubber catheter can be utilized. Through the lumen of the catheter a strong string, or cat-gut (about two feet in length), is passed. When the instrument is carried through the nostril to the pharynx, the end of the string is seized with forceps and brought out of the mouth. The tampon is then firmly tied to the middle of the string, and the plug pulled up behind the soft-palate and into the nostril. The two strings are now tied firmly over the upper lip. It is always necessary to hold the soft-palate forward with the index finger, so as to permit the tampon to pass behind it. The tampon should be removed in from twenty-four to forty-eight hours. Unless the patient is weak from loss of blood. the nostril should be cleansed by an antiseptic douche before applying either an anterior or a posterior plug.

Therapeutics

Aconite. Plethoric persons, blood bright red; hemorrhage brought on by excitement or passion. When this remedy is indicated, the characteristic fever, thirst and restlessness are present.

Arnica. Nose-bleed the result of concussion, strains or physical exertion. Epistaxis in low grades of fever.

Belladonna. Preceded by throbbing, congestive headache, with red face. Blood bright red. Nose-bleed in children at night.

Bryonia. Bleeding of the nose when the menses should appear. Nose-bleed, especially early in the morning. Blood bright red.

Cactus. Nose-bleed due to cardiac disturbance; palpitation of the heart; fluttering over stomach. Blood bright red.

China. When the hemorrhage has been of sufficient severity to cause great weakness. Anæmic, face pale, ringing in the ears.

Crocus. Blood dark, stringy.

Erechthites. Epistaxis of bright red blood. In plethoric subjects when headache precedes the nose-bleed. In typhoid-fever and Bright's disease; dark blood, passive hemorrhage.

Ferrum picricum, 3x trituration, is claimed to be almost a specific for epistaxis.

Hamamelis. General tendency to varicoses. Epistaxis, flow passive, dark colored blood. Nose-bleed occurring with hæmoptysis. Suppressed menstruation, dark blood from nose.

Lachesis. Nose-bleed with amenorrhœa during the climacteric. Epistaxis during low grades of fever, with great prostration.

Melilotus. The epistaxis relieves intense headaches of a periodical nature. (θ or 1x dilution.)

Millefolium. Nose-bleed in congestion of the head and chest; blood dark, or may be bright red.

Nux vomica. Nose-bleed in morning from suppressed hemorrhoidal flow. Blood bright red.

Phosphorus. Hæmorrhagic diathesis, spots of ecchymosis on the skin. Profuse long-lasting nose-bleed.

Pulsatilla. Nose-bleed with suppressed menses, blood dark and coagulated.

Secale cor. During fevers, bleeding of nose, blood dark; great prostration.

Sepia. Nose-bleed during pregnancy and with hemorrhoids. Epistaxis in young women during menses.

Trillium pen. Passive hemorrhage.

Thlaspi bursa pastoris. Epistaxis, blood dark and clotted.

Chapter V

SYPHILITIC RHINITIS

Definition. The term syphilitic rhinitis is used to define an inflammation of the nasal mucous membrane, and sometimes of the cartilages and bones of the nose, which is caused by the special virus of syphilis.

Etiology. I shall here discuss only the acquired form of syphilis. Primary syphilis in the nose is seldom seen, and when found is usually the result of the contagium being carried by the fingers, or by instruments. The secondary and tertiary stages, on the other hand, frequently implicate the mucous membrane of the upper respiratory tract.

Symptoms. The primary chancre occurs one to five weeks or more after infection. It is generally circular, its edges are elevated, and it presents a scooped out appearance; and the discharge is muco-purulent. Accompanying it there may be swelling of the tissues within the nostrils. The submaxillary and cervical glands are usually enlarged.

The secondary stage generally develops within six months, but may be postponed for a much longer period. During the early part of this stage there are no well marked nasal symptoms to distinguish the specific condition from a simple rhinitis. Occasionally a history of inoculation can be obtained, which was followed by an erythematous condition of the skin covering the chest, back or shins, or by mucous patches within the nostrils, or on the mucous membrane of the oral cavity.

The foregoing symptoms occurring during an obstinate rhinitis should be considered sufficient for diagnostic purposes.

The secondary stage may gradually merge into the tertiary, there being no clear line of distinction between the two. The virus may spend itself during the secondary stage, or it may remain dormant for forty years or longer, then suddenly show itself. The tertiary stage is characterized by blocking of the nostrils, due to infiltration of the mucous membrane; and by ulceration with offensive muco-purulent secretion, which may be slightly bloody. When this secretion dries in the nostrils it forms yellowish-green scabs. If not checked, the ulceration destroys the cartilaginous and bony septum and occasionally extends to the other bones of the face and skull. With the destruction of the septum the bridge of the nose is apt to fall in, presenting the so-called "saddle nose." Small red nodules may appear on the alæ of the nose and are usually followed by the destructive process. This, with the sunken bridge, causes frightful deformity.

When the bones become necrosed, the odor is almost unbearable to others in the room, yet the patient is unable to detect it as his sense of smell is apt to be wholly destroyed. The roughened bone can usually be felt by using the probe. The ulceration not infrequently attacks the hard palate on the floor of the nose, causing perforation; this may be small, or the destructive process may destroy the entire roof of the mouth. During the early part of this stage *gummata* may appear on the septum or the turbinals; sometimes they become elongated and resemble mucous polypi. In nearly all cases, during the second and third stages, the pharynx and larynx are involved.

Diagnosis. During the early part of the secondary stage syphilitic rhinitis cannot always be distinguished from the non-specific, unless there are present the skin eruptions and mucous patches in the mouth, or a clear history of contagion. Cases of hypertrophic rhinitis, where the turbinals resume their former enlargement after cauterization, and which are characterized, in addition, by tenderness of the nasal bones, must be looked upon with suspicion.

Malignant disease is confined to the septum of one nostril; the sub-lingual glands may be swollen, but the pharynx and larynx are not affected.

Prognosis. Provided the patient has not been mercurialized during the first stage, decided benefit can be expected in the succeeding stages with proper treatment persistently followed, unless excessive destruction of tissue has taken place. Yet cases are occasionally met with in scrofulous, or tuberculous patients, where *the destructive process cannot be stayed.*

It must be borne in mind that contraction of tissue due to syphilitic destruction is difficult, and not infrequently impossible, to overcome.

Treatment. The main reliance must be placed on the constitutional remedy, though cleanliness is necessary for the patient's comfort, and topical applications are valuable to limit ulceration.

For cleansing, the sprays and douches suggested for chronic and atrophic rhinitis are to be used. When ulceration is progressive the destructive process may be retarded by touching the edges of the ulcer with the solid stick of the nitrate of silver. Boracic acid, or aristol, thoroughly dusted over the surfaces of the ulcers, by means of a powder-blower, will also give good results. Ulcers occurring in the pharynx and larynx must be freed of all secretions by the use of an alkaline spray, or by using dry absorbent cotton, after which they are to be swabbed once a day with a ten-grain solution of nitrate of silver.

Necrosed bone in the nostrils must be removed, either by forceps or by the curette; it is never wise to wait for spiculæ of bone to be exfoliated by the process of ulceration.

All active syphilitics must be warned not to use public drinking cups, nor permit another to carry to his mouth any article which they have used, until it has been first properly washed.

For the sunken bridge, or destruction of the alæ, plastic operations will sometimes help to overcome the deformity, but when great destruction has taken place, a wax nose, held in position by a spectacle-frame, can be worn.

Due attention must be given to building up the patient's general health, by nourishing food, exercise, proper clothing, etc. All excesses must be strictly prohibited.

Therapeutics

As more or less pharyngitis and laryngitis attend syphilitic rhinitis the following indications are given to cover these complications: in acquired syphilis very few remedies are needed. The secondary stage will always develop, no matter what form of treatment was used in the first stage. If the first stage was treated by mercury in potency, the second stage is more readily controlled; but if the first stage was treated by material doses of mercury, the secondary stage will usually require some other remedy.

Mercurius sol. In the primary stage this preparation of mercury usually gives the best results. The 2x trituration a two-grain powder twice a day for two weeks should be given, then once a day for the same period, then every alternate day for two weeks. When given in this manner the succeeding stages are more easily managed.

In the secondary stage our main reliance is still to be placed on the proper preparation and use of mercury.

Mercurius bin. In scrofulous cases. Sneezing, blocking of the nose; turbinal bones swollen, with whitish-yellow, or bloody discharge; raw sensation in posterior nares; deafness; eruptions on the alæ of the nose. Swelling of tonsils and sub-maxillary glands; palate and tonsils dark red; loss of voice. It is my practice to give this drug in the 1x or 2x trituration twice a day.

Mercurius proto. Usually indicated as the secondary stage is merging into the tertiary stage. Mucous membrane livid, purple. Ulcerated spots on the posterior wall of the pharynx. Salivary glands swollen; much tenacious mucus in the throat; hoarse, husky voice; fetid discharge. I prefer this remedy in the 1x trituration.

Mercurius cor. When this preparation is called for, there is rapid destruction of tissue. Swelling and redness of the nose; rawness and burning in the nostrils; gluey discharge from the nose; the nostrils feel stopped up but still they run. Perforation of the septum. Swollen tonsils covered with ulcers; intense swelling and inflammation of the throat, threatening suffocation. Uvula swollen, elongated. dark-red and ulcerated. Liquids regurgitate through the nose. Burning, cutting pain in throat when swallowing. Cannot bear outside pressure on the throat. Secretion intensely fetid.

During the tertiary period it is advisable to give one of the mercurial preparations two or three times a day, but for the great destruction of tissue the main reliance must be placed on some form of potash.

Kali iodide. Face pale, colorless; nose red and swollen, throbbing pain or tightness in the nasal and frontal bones. Discharge from nose greenish or yellowish; *gummata* on the septum; ulceration of septum. Œdematous condition of pharynx. Intense swelling of the epiglottis; this may be so great that the vocal cords cannot be seen. Choking spells, hoarseness, cough; ulceration of cartilages. Discharge extremely fetid. Swelling of cervical gland. Nightly bone pains.

I believe this is a remedy that must be given in syphilis in material doses. I begin by giving the saturated solution, five drops in milk or water, fifteen minutes before or one hour after each meal, increasing each dose one drop a day until I see favorable results, until if necessary forty-drop doses are given. As soon as improvement begins the dose is decreased one or two drops a day until three drops are reached. Three drops three times a day is then continued every alternate week for five or six months, then the 2x trituration is given every second or third week for two years.

Aurum met., 3x trituration. Bones of the nose and face tender and painful; boring pain worse at night; nose red and swollen. Caries of nasal septal and palate bones; nose blocked with bloody mucus difficult to dislodge; ozæna. Melancholy, low-spirited, suicidal tendency. (*Aurum muriaticum* in the scrofulous or ill-nourished.)

Fluoric acid. Nightly bone pains; nose red and swollen, with ulceration of the septum; red blotches on the palate; soft palate and uvula red and tumefied. Throat dry, causing hawking; voice weak.

Kali bichrom. Small ulcers on the mucous membrane; destruction of the cartilaginous septum; edges of the ulcer covered with adherent, yellowish-green, hard scabs. Pressure at root of nose, pain extending to frontal sinuses and cheek bones. Loss of smell; frequent bleeding from the nose. Deep sores on soft palate with reddish areolæ, and tough, stringy mucus. Fauces dark-red or coppery. Rough, hoarse voice; metallic cough.

Nitric acid. Face yellow or pale, tip of nose red. Ozæna with ulcers; offensive, yellow mucus; nose bleeds on slightest touch. Ulcers on corners of the mouth; teeth sensitive, tongue and gums sore; the gums bleed easily. Pricking as from a splinter in the throat, worse when swallowing. Hoarseness, with scratching in the throat. Condylomata on the mucous membranes. Overdosed with mercury. When used in low potency should be freshly prepared at frequent intervals.

Phytolacca. Pain in face and head bones at night; drawing sensation in the root of the nose. Swelling of sub-lingual glands; ulcers on tonsils and soft palate; throat sore, dark red, burning, smarting; feels as though a plug were in the throat. Loss of voice.

CHAPTER VI

TUMORS OF THE NOSE

Tumors of the nose may be benign or malignant.

Of benign, the *mucous polypus* is the variety most frequently found. The *papillomata, angiomata* and polypoidal cysts were occasionally met with.

Malignant tumors in the nasal cavities are of decidedly infrequent occurrence. They include *sarcoma, carcinoma* and *epithelioma*.

NASAL POLYPUS

Synonyms. Mucous polyp. Gelatinous polyp.

Etiology. In all cases presenting these growths there is present an abnormal condition of the nasal cavities, there being always some degree of hypertrophic rhinitis.

The theory has been advanced that, owing to some impairment of the circulation in the nasal vessels, an œdematous condition of the membrane results. This, aided by gravity, and the irritation caused by blowing the nose, causes the membrane gradually to sag down, and, becoming filled with serum, drags on its attachment, thus giving the peculiar pear-shape so frequently developed. This explanation is sufficient to account for the existence of polypi on the free borders of the turbinals, but not when they occur on the outer wall of the nostril. Not infrequently there is co-existing deflection of the septal cartilage, with spurs or ridges on the septum. In many cases there is present empyema of the maxillary sinus, disease of the ethmoid cells or of the frontal sinuses. Woakes claims that a polypus is only a symptom of ethmoid bone disease. His theory has been strongly controverted by others, who contend that the bone necrosis is a result of the tumors. From the fact that polypi frequently exist with disease of the ethmoid bone, and that necrosis of the ethmoid bone may not be accompanied by polypi, it is evident that neither is necessarily a cause of the other. In the first case, a mass of polypi wedged in between the septum and middle turbinal, by the pressure exerted, causes inflammation, the vitality of the bone becoming impaired and ending in necrosis. As to the claim advanced by Woakes, it can readily be seen that a primary necrosis in the ethmoid spongy bone, with its resulting purulent discharge, may so affect the mucous membrane as to cause it to become swollen, sacculated, and thus result in formation of a polypus or polypi; a condition analogous to aural polypus the result of otitis media with necrosis. Any frequent irritation extending over a prolonged period of time may also produce polypi. I have seen several cases where the patient was in the habit of making applications of patent medicine cerates—by means of a lead pencil—to the nasal cavities. The irritation thus caused was evidently a strong factor in the formation of the tumors.

The growths are usually attached to the middle turbinal or to the middle meatus. When growing from the lower turbinal they have a broader base of attachment. Occasionally they spring from the septum.

Nasal polypi are almost invariably multiple; it is rare to find a case with only one polypus; but usually one side contains more tumors than the other. Nasal polypi are somewhat more frequent in the male sex. The majority of cases are over twenty years of age, yet they are sometimes seen in children.

In some families there appears to be an hereditary tendency to polypus formation on the mucous surfaces.

Diagnosis. Ordinarily, with the aid of a reflector, a proper light and a nasal speculum, the diagnosis is not difficult. Their color is usually of a grayish-white, or somewhat resembling the pulp of a grape or of an oyster. Tumors of a pale, pinkish color are occasionally seen. From other forms of tumors they are to be distinguished by their freedom from pain and non-vascularity. Under the application of cocaine hypertrophy of the turbinals will decrease, whereas on mucous polypi the drug has no depletory effect. Cartilaginous and bony tumors of the septum are hard, and not displaced by pressure. Fibrous tumors are more solid, of a pink color, and frequently excite epistaxis. Malignant tumors are decidedly vascular, tend to ulceration with an ichorous, fetid discharge, and the characteristic pain common to malignant tumors is rarely absent. The varicose enlargement on the posterior ends of the lower turbinals are to be distinguished from mucous polypi by their location, darker color, and usually raspberry-like surface. In hypertrophic rhinitis the anterior end of the lower turbinal, and the free border of the middle turbinal, frequently present a light color much resembling mucous polypi, but have a broader base of attachment, and shrink under the action of cocaine; this condition is not a tumor, but hypertrophy of the mucous membrane and sub-mucous tissues.

Symptoms. The symptoms necessarily depend on the number and the size of the polypi. The patient first notices a sense of obstruction in the nostrils; this stuffiness is increased during damp weather. The aggravation during damp weather is probably due to the action of humidity on the accompanying rhinitis which is present, and not to hygroscopic properties of the polypi. In uncomplicated nasal polypi the discharge is invariably semi-transparent, grayish, and watery in character; but where there is co-existing disease of the accessory sinuses the discharge is yellowish or purulent and the patient complains of an offensive discharge in the back of the mouth, and in the throat, which is worse in the morning. When a polypus is attached to the border of the middle turbinal it may give the sensation of a valve-like motion during forced nasal breathing.

The sense of smell, and frequently of taste, as well, is impaired or destroyed. When smell is not wholly lacking the patient may complain of a mousy or musty odor. Sneezing is frequent, more especially so if the posterior half of the nostrils s implicated.

As the tumors increase in number and size, frontal headache, deafness and ocular disturbances are common. Reflex neurcses frequently result, perhaps the most frequent being asthma and cough. The voice is indicative of the nasal lesion. It has been described as "a dead voice with a faint nasal tone to it."

Mucous polypi rarely if ever cause external deformity of the nose, unless they make their appearance during childhood and are not removed early. The upper part of the nose may appear broader than normal, but this is due to venous congestion, with resulting œdema. Nor do polypi cause a deflection of the septum. When the foregoing deformities are present, they are due to prior causes and probably are a local factor in the tendency to formation of polypi.

A yellow, muco-purulent or purulent discharge may be present, and if there is occasional pain with a sense of fulness or tightness over the region of the maxillary or ethmoidal cavities, it is quite conclusive that empyema of one or both cavities exists. This condition is caused by the tumors growing from, or occluding the orifices of the accessory sinuses, thus preventing access of air to the cavity; their normal secretion is retained, and inflammation, terminating in suppuration, results.

In polypi, as in all other forms of nasal stenosis, the pharynx is implicated to some extent.

Prognosis. Uncomplicated mucous polypi involve no danger to life, but when so situated as to interfere with æration of accessory sinuses and to cause mouth breathing, serious complications may result. It has been claimed that malignant degeneration has followed removal of mucous polypi, but it is a question whether such degeneration can occur. In the cases so reported it is more probable that an error was made in the first diagnosis, or that a benign and a malignant tumor co-existed. A few weeks after the removal of the polypi new tumors may occupy the same space. Whether these spring from the point of attachment of former tumors not thoroughly removed, or from the adjacent mucous membrane, is an unsettled question.

When the polypi are complicated with disease of the sinuses, recurrences may be expected until the sinus disease is relieved.

Treatment. This consists in surgical removal or cauterization of the growths, and the local application of astringent drugs. In addition all cases demand a careful selection of the constitutional remedy. Experience teaches that to proper local and internal treatment the best results follow. Neither one should be used to the exclusion of the other. The various acids and astringents used for injecting polypi need to be mentioned only to be condemned.

The recognized surgical means of removal are: avulsion with the forceps; abscission with the cold wire snare; and galvano or chemical cauterizaton.

Before operatng, a four per cent. solution of cocaine should be applied. This not only renders the operation painless, but depletes the surrounding tissue, thereby obtaining larger space for the use of the instruments. Operations within the nostrils should not be performed without the use of a proper light and the aid of a nasal speculum. Blind operation is an injury, not a benefit.

Avulsion, by tearing the tumor off with forceps, is to be used only when the growth cannot be encircled with the wire loop of a snare. The main objection to the forceps is the liability of causing pain and bleeding by tearing the surrounding mucous membrane.

Abscission, with the Bosworth or Sajous snare, is the most satisfactory method of removal. The wire loop is made to encircle the tumor and is then carried to its point of attachment, when by quickly tightening the wire the growth is cut off.

The galvano-cautery snare may be used, but it is more difficult of manipulation, and possesses no advantages over the cold wire.

If the growths are small, they may be destroyed by touching them with acid, or the galvano-cautery point.

After the cavities are cleared, it is advisable to cauterize with acid, or, preferably, the electric cautery, any remaining polypoid tissue.

At least once a month for a year after removal of the tumors, the nostrils should be examined for recurrence of the growths. If at the end of that time the nostrils are free, the case can be considered cured.

Therapeutics

The selection of the internal remedy—when empyema of the sinuses is not a complication—depends more on the general symptoms presented, than on the local indications. However, a choice can usually be made from one of the following:

Calcarea carb., *Calcarea phos.*, *Hydrastis*, *Kali bich.*, *Kali nit.*, *Nitric acid*, *Phosphorus*, *Sanguinaria Can.*, *Staphisagria*, *Teucrium* and *Thuja*.

Consult Chronic Rhinitis, and Diseases of the Accessory Sinuses.

PAPILLOMATA

Etiology. The cause of papillomata or warty growths occurring in the nostrils, is not known. But as papillomata growing on other mucous membranes of the body are frequently due to irritation, it is reasonable to infer that the same cause may be a factor in exciting similar growths of the nasal passages.

Diagnosis. These growths usually first appear between puberty and middle life. They are, invariably, attached to the septum, or to the free border of the lower turbinals. When presenting near the external nasal orifice, their shape and size are similar to the cutaneous wart.

But when occurring further back in the nostril they are of a deep pink color, are larger in size, and of a more irregular surface. They are attached to the mucous membrane by a broad base, and rarely attain a size larger than a small raspberry. More often they are about the size of a split pea.

Symptoms. These growths—when unattended by other nasal lesions—give rise to no distinctive symptoms. Bleeding may be frequent; and if the tumor increases in size, stenosis of the affected nostril will be present.

Prognosis. The prognosis is favorable.

Treatment. They should be removed by means of the galvano-cautery, snare, or by the cold wire loop. The application of chromic acid, or nitric acid, will destroy them.

Internally, *Thuja oc*. is the chief remedy, especially if the growth shows a tendency to recur after surgical removal.

CYSTS

Cystic tumors in the nasal cavities are of rare occurrence. Their appearance is similar to a mucous polypus. Their removal is easily accomplished by means of a cold wire snare. When the enveloping membrane is torn a watery fluid escapes, causing the tumor to collapse.

CHONDROMATA

Definition. Nasal chondromata are cartilaginous tumors, growing from the triangular cartilage of the septum, or from the inner surface of the lateral cartilages.

Etiology. The cause of these growths is unknown;

their period of development is a few years before, or, soon after, puberty.

Symptoms. This form of tumor presents no characteristic symptoms. As a result of the stenosis, or of the tumor impinging on the opposite surface, there may be present the symptoms usually found in other forms of benign growths, namely, inability to properly breathe with the affected nostril, offensive muco-purulent discharge and epistaxis. Headache and ocular disturbances may be present. If not removed, the tumor may so increase in size as to cause marked deformity of the outer wall of the nose.

Diagnosis. Nasal chondromata are round or oval in shape, presenting an irregular surface of the color of the surrounding mucous membrane. They are to be distinguished from deflections, or deformities of the nasal septum, which always present a concavity on the opposite septal wall. Chondromata usually occur at the juncture of the septal and lateral cartilages; deflections occur nearer the center of the septal cartilage.

Chondromata may be punctured with a strong needle; osteomata cannot be so pierced, and always grow from bone, or from one of the accessory cavities.

Prognosis. The growth is not prone to recur after removal.

Treatment. They can be sawed off, or they may be pared off with a sharp bistoury.

OSTEOMATA

Nasal osteomata are a rare form of bony tumor growing from accessory cavities, or more rarely from the upper part of the nostrils.

They more frequently occur in the male at about the twentieth year of age. There are two varieties, the more common being the dense growth resembling ivory or marble in its hardness; and the softer, composed largely of cancellous structure. They are somewhat pedunculated; their point of attachment is probably the periosteum.

Owing to the obstruction, and irritation due to friction, there results a fetid muco-purulent, or bloody discharge. When not removed, their tendency is constantly to increase in size; this may progress to the extent of causing great facial deformity.

There is constant neuralgic pain, intense headache, and sometimes, displacement of the eye-ball.

Fortunately this form of tumor is extremely rare. When seen before serious changes have occurred, the prognosis is favorable.

When small, removal is accomplished by severing the pedicle by the means of the saw, or strong cutting forceps. When of considerable size, the trephine or drill may be used.

Although I have never seen a nasal tumor of this character it occurs to me that, by means of the electric trephine, the tumor could be so perforated as to permit it to be readily crushed with forceps.

MALIGNANT TUMORS OF THE NOSE SARCOMA AND CARCINOMA

Etiology. Few, if any, diseases have been more thoroughly investigated to ascertain the histogenetic cause than malignant tumors. Many theories, and frequently well substantiated, have been advanced, only to be disproven by other investigators.

The claim has been made that ulceration the result of syphilis may be an exciting cause, but such claims are not sustained by clinical experience. Among the other causes set forth are, the parasitic nature of the disease; its direct or indirect contagiousness; its hereditary tendency or its transmissibility. Traumatism and long continued irritation is undoubtedly an exciting factor. Aside from the latter cause, the conclusion must be reached that the etiology of the cancer is undetermined.

Symptoms. Primary malignant tumors in the nose usually grow from the septum, or from the middle turbinal. Secondary tumors extend from the accessory cavities or from the orbit.

In sarcoma, age is not a predisposing factor, as the majority of cases reported were seen prior to the age of forty, and cases have occurred in children, thus differing from cancer, which develops later in life. As sarcoma develops, deformity of the face ensues, due to expansion and external pressure by the growth.

In all malignant nasal tumors, epistaxis is an early and frequently recurring symptom; in sarcoma the bleeding is from ulceration of the surrounding tissue, whereas in carcer hemorrhage is due to ulceration of the growth. In both forms of tumor there is a muco-sanguinolent discharge from the affected nostril. Headache and neuralgic pains are present; but nasal cancer rarely has the intense pain so frequently accompanying cancer in other parts of the body.

In nasal sarcoma, in a certain per cent. of the cases, the cervical glands are never enlarged.

Sarcoma first presents a bluish color on the diseased

surface; cancer resembles a wart of a purple or red color.

Diagnosis. When in doubt as to the character of the growth, a small piece should be removed and submitted to microscopic examination. It is usually advisable to submit different parts of the tumor for examination, as one section may show only innocent cells, while another may show malignant growths. Yet in forming a diagnosis, the gross appearарnrce and the clinical history of the growth must be considered.

Prognosis. The prognosis necessarily depends on the age of the patient; the character, location and duration of the tumor.

The small round-cell sarcoma is not prone to recur after removal, thus differing from the spindle-cell growths, which are of a more malignant nature.

Cancer in the nose, as in other parts of the body, is exceedingly grave. When occurring in advanced life, its course is rapid, usually terminating fatally within a year. When the cancer occurs before middle life, if the character of growth is recognized before the tumor has implicated the surrounding tissue, then the prognosis is more favorable.

Treatment. In nasal sarcoma a thorough removal of the growth should be undertaken as soon as possible, and if this can be done, preferably through the nasal passage. If the nostril does not possess sufficient space in which to operate, the upper lip and infra-nasal tissues may be freed from the superior maxillary, the lip and lower part of the nose everted and drawn upward, thus affording free access to the nostrils.

As each case must be dealt with according to the

existing conditions, no one procedure can be followed in all cases.

For removing the tumor it may be necessary to use the knife, saw, curette, cold wire snare, or the hot platinum loop. The main point to bear in mind is *total extirpation.*

Unless the tumor has invaded the accessory sinuses or implicated the surrounding tissues, cocaine anæsthesia, when operating through the natural passages, is sufficient.

Bleeding during the operation is quite profuse, but ceases almost entirely after removal of the growth.

In regard to nasal carcinoma, it is the generally accepted opinion that surgical treatment, unless begun before the surrounding tissue is implicated, does not retard but rather hastens a fatal issue.

In such cases the utmost that can be accomplished is a possible retardation of the inevitable fatality and, to modify the pain.

An injection of a thirty per cent. solution of lactic acid into the tumor has been alleged to arrest the growth of sarcoma.

The daily hypodermic injection of tannin, one part, to glycerine twenty-four parts, is recommended. Alveloz juice locally has been claimed to cure cancer.

The special toxine of erysipelas in combination with the toxins of bacillus prodigiosus, injected into the tumor, is said to have cured a few cases of cancer; whether it has been used in cancer of the nose and with what result I am unable to learn.

A constantly applied local application of acetic acid No. 8, two per cent. solution, combined with the internal administration of a four to ten per cent. solution, four or five times a day has, it is claimed, cured tumors having the appearance of carcinoma. Daily applications of resorcin and vaseline, equal parts, applied to malignant tumors is credited with curative results.

Comfort will frequently be derived from the use of sprays containing morphine, belladonna, calendula or cocaine. When the latter is used, it is necessary frequently to increase the strength of the solution.

In a disease where the pain is intense and death a matter of only a few weeks or months, any means that will alleviate the suffering is justifiable.

Therapeutics

There is no question that potentized remedies do frequently have more or less influence in controlling the pains of cancer. It is to be regretted, however, that the clinical cases of cancer reported in our journals as relieved or cured by internal remedies, fail to give the variety of malignant growths diagnosed. More care in diagnosing and reporting these cases would greatly aid in treating subsequent cases, and result in greater confidence in our branch of therapeutics.

A choice can usually be made from one of the following remedies: *Acetic acid*, *Aurum*, *Arsenicum*, *Belladonna*, *Carbolic acid*, *Chian turpentine*, *Conium*, *Condurango*, *Hydrastis Can.*, *Hydrocotyle Asiatica*, *Kali cyanicum*, *Kreosote*, *Galium aperinum*, *Lapis albus*, *Nitric acid*, *Phosphorus*, *Phytolacca*, *Thuja*.

Chapter VII

DEFORMITIES AND DISEASES OF THE NASAL SEPTUM

(DEVIATION OF THE SEPTUM)

Etiology. Deformity of the nasal septum is one of the most frequent conditions for which rhinologists are consulted. In fact, the majority of adults present some degree of septal deviation, although in many cases the abnormal condition is not sufficiently pronounced to demand surgical treatment.

It is generally admitted, that in the majority of cases the cause of deviation of the nasal septum is obscure.

Zuckerkandle claims, as the result of extended observation, that prior to the seventh year, the septum is always straight. But clinical experience does not verify this absolute declaration. Among the causes advanced are: the rapid growth of the septal cartilage, as compared with surrounding bones; also when a highly arched hard palate crowds the septum upward so it cannot maintain its vertical position, to accommodate the increasing growth of the septal cartilage, then deviation results.

But by far the most common cause is traumatism. The injury may occur during the passage of the child through the parturient canal. During the age of babyhood and childhood, few children escape falls, or blows, on the nose and at the time little attention may be given the accident. As stated by Bosworth, "An injury to the nose need not necessarily give rise to immediate development of a notable deformity, as in a fracture, but it may set up a low grade of morbid action, which going on through a number of years, will finally develop a condition by which the normal function of the nose is hampered * * * in such a way as to cause a low grade of inflammatory action." This abnormal condition, and the accompanying rhinitis, gradually increasing, will in the course of a few years develop either deviation of the septum or spurs and ridges on the septal walls.

As facial characteristics, and nasal contour are frequently transmitted, so I believe the same rule holds good when applied to the nasal septum.

Symptoms. The subjective symptoms are similar to those enumerated under "Hypertrophic Rhinitis."

During the act of inspiration nasal stenosis is usual on the side of the septal convexity; the ala of the affected nostril sinks in, which further prevents the entrance of air into the nostrils.

Nasal secretion is increased and drops posteriorly; neuralgic pains over the brow are frequent; complaint is made of pressure, and fulness on the affected side. Sneezing is frequent, hay-fever and asthma are reflex conditions sometimes occurring. Hearing is often less than normal. The voice is impaired, the tone is much the same as developed in other forms of nasal blocking. Dryness and crusts are present, and to relieve this irritation the patient picks and rubs the part, which often results in epistaxis, and not infrequently in ulceration. Cases are often seen where this ulcerated condition has existed for years. Pharyngeal and laryngeal irritations are usually present.

Owing to inability to properly breathe through the nostril, the inhaled air passes through the buccal cavity causing it to become dry. This is especially so in persons required to speak in public, the dryness necessitating frequent sips of water to moisten the mouth and throat.

Diagnosis. Deformities of the septum are readily recognized by means of a nasal speculum and good light. Deflections present a concavity on one side, with a corresponding convexity on the opposite wall. Nasal polypi are movable and present a lighter color than the septum. When deformity is the result of fracture the deflected part is usually thickened on both sides. To permit a thorough examination both nostrils should be anæsthetized with cocaine.

Prognosis. Increased breathing space can be assured in, probably, all cases. It is often surprising how quickly malaise, headache, cough and many of the reflex irritations are relieved by removing contact of the opposite surfaces of the nose. Tinnitus and deafness are frequently benefited, but when these conditions exist it is usually necessary to direct the treatment to the pharynx and eustachian tubes, also with a view to reducing the accompanying chronic inflammatory conditions.

Treatment. The varieties of deflections, septal spurs and ridges are so numerous that no set rule for treatment can be given. It must necessarily depend upon the conditions existing in the case at hand.

When the lower turbinal in the freer nostril is hypertrophied, it must first be reduced.

For deviation of the cartilage, the method of Adams is frequently used. This consists in introducing one blade of Adams's forceps into each nostril, and exerting sufficient pressure to force the septum into place. It is then held in position by means of ivory plugs, or steel plates, until the cure is complete. These supports are removed every day or two and the nostril cleansed.

Excision of the prominent part of the cartilage may be accomplished with a knife, saw or trephine. This method is frequently necessary when the cartilage is thickened. After the cartilage is restored to a normal condition the septum should be incised and replaced.

For removing the angular portion, Blandin's or Steele's punch-forceps may be employed. They are supplied with a variety of stellate, oval and straight blades, for the purpose of making incisions in the cartilage. Incisions thus made make it pliable and permit it to be replaced to the median line.

After the use of these punches great care is necessary to keep the parts clean, as crusts quickly form and sloughing may occur.

Another operation described consists in dissecting up the mucous membrane on the prominent part, excising a piece of the deflected cartilage, and subsequently replacing the flaps, which are held in position by sutures. This method of operating I have never tried, as I do not believe it a practical procedure. The increased breathing space obtained is no greater than is obtained in slicing off the mucous membrane and cartilage. In the latter operation, if the parts are kept in an aseptic condition, the cut surface quickly heals over and the mucous membrane readily reforms.

An operation first described by Asch frequently gives good results.

"The operation is easy to perform; it takes but a short time and does not require tedious dissection of the mucous membrane. The instruments required are a pair of cutting-forceps or scissors with a dull, concave blade on one side, and a convex cutting blade on the other, an elevator or chisel to break up any adhesions that may exist between the septum and the inferior turbinated body, and a hard rubber tubular splint of proper size, perforated at the sides, in order to enable it to retain its position and prevent slipping out. The mode of operation is as follows: the patient having been etherized, and the head drawn over the edge of the table, so as to prevent the blood from running into the larynx, and the nostrils having been sprayed with an antiseptic solution, the dull blade of the scissors is introduced into the obstructed nostril in such a direction as to permit a crucial incision to be made, the first cut being in a line parallel with the upper lip, and the second as nearly at right angles to it as the conformation of the nose will allow. These two cuts make four triangular segments. The forefinger is then introduced into the nostril on the side in which the septum projects, and the segments are bent back into the other nostril and fractured at their base.

With an Adams or any similar forceps the whole of the septum is then broken up; and the bleeding checked by spraying with cold Dobell's solution, and the tubular splint introduced into the previously obstructed nostril, where it is allowed to remain for forty-eight hours without removal, the nose being in the meantime sprayed several times a day with an antiseptic solution. After the wound has healed the patient can be allowed to introduce and remove the splint, which should be worn two or three months. It causes no discomfort if the septum has been sufficiently broken."

Asch states in no case has he seen reaction of an unfavorable kind. For controlling hemorrhage he uses an ice-cold spray and has never seen a secondary hemorrhage.

The operation that has given me the best results consists in making an incision, with a sharp-pointed bistoury, through the whole length of the prominent part of the deflected cartilage. In some cases it will be necessary to make a parallel, or a vertical incision, to reduce the resiliency of the cartilage. Then by means of the little finger, or flat forceps, carried into the obstructed side, the septum is pressed over into place with the cut edges slightly overlapping each other. After thorough cleansing it is necessary to maintain the septum in place. This can be done by packing the obstructed nostril with antiseptic gauze. Or, what is better still, tubular cork splints, as suggested by Berens. In the latter method a piece of cork, of sufficient size and shape to snugly fit in the nostril, is selected. The outer and inner surfaces of the cork are thickly coated with collodion containing thirty per cent of iodoform; the outer surface is coated with cerate, when it is inserted into the nostril. This serves to keep the septum in its new position. The operator should attend to the removal of the splint and cleansing the cavities every other day, for ten days or two weeks, after which the patient can be taught to remove and replace the splint without the aid of the physician. The splint should be used for fully six weeks, or until the septum is thoroughly healed and remains in its new position. Any inequalities of cartilage resulting can be trimmed off with a knife or scissors.

Osseous and osseo-cartilaginous spurs, or ridges, situated posteriorly to the deflection in the occluded nostril, are to be removed after straightening the cartilage. (*vide* Hypertrophic Rhinitis.)

When using the saw the cutting should, if possible, be in an upward direction, in order to prevent the blood concealing the portion to be removed, as would be the case when the cutting is from above downward.

The stronger acids, such as nitric, or chromic, should never be applied to the septum; and in using the galvano-cautery deep incisions must be avoided, as frequently the cartilage does not heal kindly after its use and tends to ulceration.

As a rule, cocaine solution, thoroughly applied on each side of the septum, is the only anæsthetic required.

During, or as a result of, the cutting operations perforation of the septum may occur. This is not a serious matter; in fact, it is often of benefit, if breathing space is required. Usually the edges of the opening heal kindly, if proper after-treatment is followed.

PERFORATION OF THE SEPTUM

Etiology. Perforation of the septum may be due to a variety of causes, such as perichondritis, the result of traumatism, or abscess. The inhalation of the fumes of chromic acid may also cause perforation of the cartilage. Lowered vitality, and septic conditions, as tuberculosis, diphtheria, and typhoid fever may produce it. Perforation of the cartilage, the result of epistaxis, is not infrequent in scrofulous patients.

An opening through the cartilage of the septum is often due to picking the nose to remove adhered crusts and scabs in atrophic rhinitis; or to the irritation caused by a deformed septum in contact with the opposite wall.

Perforation caused by syphilis is always accompanied by fetor, the result of necrosis of some part of the bony frame-work.

Treatment. Any underlying dyscrasia should receive proper constitutional treatment. A generous nutritious diet, and proper exercise are essential; in fact, all means should be used tending to build up the general health.

Cleansing local applications, to keep the parts free from crust, should be used. For this purpose alkaline douches followed by calendula, or hamamelis cerates; or five to fifteen grains of yellow oxide of mercury, to one ounce of lanoline; or fresh lard, applied morning and night to the denuded edges, are useful.

Perforation of the septum never closes. The whole cartilage may be destroyed without any falling-in of the nose. The bridge of the nose will become sunken only when due to syphilis, or when the nasal bones are diseased. This latter condition may be restored by proper plastic operations.

HÆMATOMA

As a result of injury, extravasation of blood may take place on the septum. The tumor presents a bluish or purplish color.

There is frequent œdema of the external parts, the swelling extending to the loose tissues around the eye, and to the cheek.

Treatment consists in aspiration, or making a small incision in the most dependent part of the tumor.

ABSCESS

Abscess of the septum may be due to perichondritis; or may result from hæmatoma. Local pain, swelling and redness of the nose attend the formation of pus. Increased pulse and temperature may be present.

Syphilitic gummata on the septum may resemble abscess, but the history of the case, and other symptoms present, make the diagnosis clear.

The treatment is surgical.

A free incision to permit the pus to escape should be made. When the perichondrium is implicated it may be necessary to curette the cavity.

Chapter VIII

FOREIGN BODIES IN THE NOSE

Etiology. Children not infrequently insert various foreign bodies into the nostril. Commonly it is a shoe button, bean, small pebble, piece of slate pencil, or a hair-pin. Hysterical women and insane persons often have the same habit. Among the rarer causes is the accidental lodging of solid substances ejected from the stomach during the act of vomiting, the force with which the contents of the stomach are ejected causing the body to enter the nostrils posteriorly. If too large to pass through it may become impacted.

Symptoms. In a child, a unilateral nasal discharge of a muco-purulent, or bloody character, is sufficient cause for making an examination for a foreign body. Through timidity, or fright, the child may deny inserting any substance into the nostril. Beans and peas absorb the watery secretion in the nostril, thus causing them to swell, which gives rise to considerable pain.

I once saw a case where a boy inserted a dry strip of leather into the nose, which in the course of a week, became thoroughly water-soaked; the expansion of the leather, and consequent inflammation, caused decided swelling of the nose and cheek.

Epistaxis is common when the substance is rough or sharp-pointed. Obstruction, sneezing, loss of smell, and pain of a neuralgic character are often present, these several symptoms varying with the size and character of the body. It is usually impacted between the lower, or middle turbinal and the septum.

Diagnosis. Rarely can reliance be placed on the history of these cases. Not infrequently is it suspected that a child has inserted something in the nose when such is not the case; on the other hand, a foreign body may remain in the nose for years without being suspected.

When the patient can be controlled, a thorough examination should be made with the aid of reflected light. The mucous membrane may become so swollen as completely to hide the offending body. When such is the case, the application of cocaine will usually deplete the tissues so the foreign body can be detected with the probe.

Harsh treatment is wholly unnecessary; it is liable to cause bleeding, and thus increase the difficulty in diagnosing and removing the body.

Prognosis. The prognosis is generally favorable. Perforation of the septum is an occasional result of tightly impacted bodies; but the ulceration readily yields to local treatment.

Treatment. In the case of children it is better to give a general anæsthetic in order to avoid injuring the mucous membrane, which would be likely to occur if the child is held.

After locating, and determining the size of the foreign body, it can usually be seized and extracted with a pair of forceps, care being taken not to include any of the soft tissue. The use of snares, probangs, and douches is questionable, as they are liable to cause injury, which can be avoided by careful manipulation of the forceps.

RHINOLITHS

Synonyms. Nasal calculi. Nasal stone.

Etiology. Occasionally a foreign body remaining in the nostril for some time, becomes encrusted with a deposit of carbonate, or phosphate of lime from the nasal secretions. Or the nucleus of a rhinolith may be a hardened piece of mucus, blood-clot, or spiculæ of bone.

Symptoms. The symptoms produced by a rhinolith are the same as those caused by any other foreign body in the nose; the degree of obstruction, discharge, pain, etc., varying with the size and location of the calcareous body. As it usually requires years for the calculus to form, the majority of cases are met with in adults.

Diagnosis. After the nostril is thoroughly cocainized, a careful examination with the probe, will detect a hard or gritty surface. The only disease with which it may be confounded is roughened bone, the result of syphilis. In the latter disease, however, other confirmatory symptoms are present.

Prognosis. The prognosis is favorable. The granulations and discharge speedily yield to mild local treatment.

If distortion of the nasal bones is present, they may require subsequent operations to correct the deformity.

Treatment. If the rhinolith is small, the same method of removal as directed under "Foreign Bodies in the Nose," will usually prove sufficient. If large, the calculus may have to be crushed with forceps; or if extremely hard, a lithotrite may be necessary. This should always be done under a general anæsthetic, the operator guarding against undue injury to the surrounding tissue.

PARASITES IN THE NOSE

In the temperate zone, parasites in the nose are very

rare, but cases are reported where ascarides, ear-wings, leeches, and cimices, have been found in the nostrils; also flies may enter the nostrils, deposit their ova, and maggots result.

In the tropics a disease known as "Peenash" is quite common. It is caused by maggots gaining entrance into the nose, and not infrequently into the nasal sinuses. As the disease progresses, inflammation, and ulceration resulting in caries and terminating in meningitis causing death, is not uncommon.

Treatment by inhalations of chloroform: nasal douche of equal parts of chloroform and water, also injections of diluted alcohol, will usually be sufficient to destroy the parasites.

Chapter IX

PERIODICAL HYPERESTHETIC RHINITIS

Synonyms. Hay-fever. Rose cold. Pollen catarrh. Peach cold. Autumnal catarrh.

Definition. Hay-fever may be designated as a recurring summer or autumnal attack of acute rhinitis, with implication of the conjunctivæ, and frequently with paroxysms of asthma, in susceptible individuals; caused by certain pollen or emanations in the atmosphere.

Etiology. As all in same locality are subject to the same exciting conditions that cause periodic acute catarrh in some, there must be certain individual conditions present. The necessary factors for the production of hay-fever as advanced by Sajous, and now accepted by most rhinologists, are:

First. A predisposing constitutional condition.

Second. A pathological condition of the nasal mucous membrane.

Third. The external irritant.

The absence of any one of these conditions is sufficient to prevent an attack.

What the predisposing constitutional condition is it is not always possible to determine. As the same plant does not reach the same stage, at the same hour or day each year, the periodicity can only be accounted for by the individual's anticipation of the attack. This psychical influence is well illustrated by Mackenzie, who records a case where an attack of hay-fever was precipitated by the patient looking upon a picture of a field of hay. According to carefully collected statistics, in one-fifth of all cases, more than one member of the same family were affected.

In all cases an abnormal pathological condition of the mucous membrane of the nose, or naso-pharynx, is present; this may be manifest by hypertrophy of the turbinals, more especially the posterior two-thirds of the lower and the middle turbinals; sub-mucous swelling on the posterior borders of the septum; cartilaginous, or bony spurs, or ridges on the septum, or deflection of the same. In many cases mucous polypi are present, but it is a question whether the polypi constitute one of the causes, or are a result of the annual catarrh. In the posterior nares there is frequently present a degree of pharyngeal hypertrophy accompanied by enlargement of the follicles. It is not unusual to find elongation of the uvula, and chronic hypertrophy of the faucial tonsils.

The external irritant is the pollen from certain grasses, weeds, flowers, or fruit, *i.e.*, timothy hay, ragweed, golden-rod, nasturtiums, June roses, peach skin, etc. In the lake region, the attack usually occurs when the grapes are turning purple or blue, about the middle of August. Flowers and grasses are more likely to cause an attack when dried or cut, than when green. All hay-fever sufferers are not susceptible to the action of pollen from the same plants. During the hay-fever season, the emanations from the horse or cat will frequently provoke an attack.

Most authors claim that hay-fever is more prevalent in cities than in the country districts. To this I cannot agree; having had a somewhat extended experience, in both city and country practice, I believe that in a given population there is a larger per cent. of cases of hay-fever in the country than in the city. The rural sufferer is not as likely to consult a physician for this disease as his city brother, hence the apparent freedom in the country.

Symptoms. Often the individual who has passed through several sieges will foretell exactly the day and the hour of the attack. A frequent premonitory warning, occurring two or three days in advance, is a sense of itching of the roof of the mouth and the inner canthi.

In the beginning the symptoms are similar to those of acute rhinitis. Itching in the nose and roof of the mouth; sneezing, which is frequently paroxysmal; free watery discharge, swelling of the nasal lining membranes, which causes blocking of the nostrils, and which may increase so that breathing through the nostrils is impossible. There is present itching and burning sensation of the conjunctivæ, followed by lachrymation. Owing to its acrid character, the watery discharge soon excoriates the skin with which it comes in contact. During the early stage, chilliness followed by fever, malaise, severe frontal headache, pain in the eyeballs, loss of the sense of smell and taste is common.

As the disease progresses the earlier conditions become greatly intensified. Tinnitus aurium with some degree of deafness is present. The larynx and bronchial tubes become involved. With this condition the paroxysms of asthma begin, and make their appearance earlier each succeeding year.

The nasal and conjunctival irritations are worse during the daytime, and in the bright sunlight, frequently becoming so intense that the patient seeks the seclusion of a darkened room. The asthmatic attacks are invariably harder at night, passing off somewhat before daybreak. During rainy summers the hay-fever sieges are usually milder, due, no doubt, to the lessened quantity of pollen floating in the atmosphere.

Prognosis. The rose-cold beginning during May and June usually terminates during the early part of August. But the true hay-fever attacks that begin during August, unless relieved by treatment or by removal to a locality exempt from hay-fever, continues until the first heavy or black frost, which, in this climate, occurs early in November.

Provided thorough and intelligent local treatment is instituted, followed by careful selection of the constitutional remedy, the majority of cases can be cured, and nearly all can be relieved, but to accomplish this may require yearly treatment for two or three years. Hay-fever patients are proverbial for desiring to change physicians each year. The greater the pathological condition presented during the intervals, usually the more favorable will be the result. In individuals past the half century mile-stone, the prognosis will be less hopeful.

After the disease has subsided, the patient is often left in a debilitated condition, from which he may not recover for weeks or months.

Treatment. During the intervals of the attacks, the nostrils should receive careful attention; all existing pathological conditions, such as mucous polypi, spurs or ridges on the septum, enlargement of the turbinals, special attention being given to the posterior third of the lower and middle turbinals, and the corresponding surface of the septum, and puffy œdematous, and sensitive areas on the septum, must be removed; when contact exists between the middle turbinal and the septum, sufficient of the former must be removed to prevent its impinging on the septal wall. The method of treatment followed should be the same as directed under "Hypertrophic Rhinitis," and "Diseases of the Septum."

Proper diet, exercise and rest must be insisted on, and no sluggishness of the bowels or constipation permitted.

When the individual seeks relief during the attack, some form of local palliative treatment may be employed; although such measures may not cure, yet we are not justified in withholding from our patient any treatment which will modify his sufferings, and yet not interfere with the constitutional remedy.

In a disease so universal it is not surprising that countless methods for obtaining temporary relief have been suggested.

Plugging the nostrils with cotton, wearing respirators and veils, so as to to prevent the entrance of pollen into the nostrils, have been used, yet the discomforts incident to the use of such methods are so great that many patients prefer the disease to the cure.

A one-half to four per cent. cocaine solution in albolene, used three or four times a day, by means of a vaporizer, will frequently mitigate the severity of the sneezing. In the use of cocaine the caution heretofore insisted on is to be remembered. Excellent results are claimed by using a five per cent spray of antipyrine; also from penciling the nasal mucous membrane with carbolic acid one part to glycerine three parts. The quinine spray is frequently recommended, this is made by dissolving one grain of quinine in an ounce and a half of water; before using the solution it is to be heated to 100° F.

Recently it has been claimed that lithæmia is a strong predisposing cause of hay-fever, and that gratifying results follow a fifteen grain dose of salicylate of soda, taken before breakfast.

Naphthalene, protoiodide of mercury, hamamelis, or belladonna ointment freely applied to the nostrils are claimed to be beneficial; favorable results have been credited to the use of hydriodic acid syrup; a pill of atropia sulphate containing the two-hundredth of a grain every three or four hours, until its physiological effect is produced (manifested by dryness in the throat and nose), will lessen an attack.

Amelioration will occasionally follow inhalation of the compound tincture of benzoin, one drachm to a pint of hot water.

Therapeutics

Aralia rac. "Extreme sensitiveness to a draught, the least current of air causing sneezing with watery, acrid discharge from nostrils and posterior nares." Nightly attacks of asthma, inability to lie down. After first sleep patient wakes with a cough, which is relieved by expectoration.

Arsenicum iod. When given in the 3x trituration, once a day, for three weeks before the expected attack, it will frequently modify the nasal irritation. Sneezing, profuse, acrid discharge from nose, excoriating border of nostrils and the upper lip. Burning and itching in nostrils and throat, and on the roof of the mouth. Frequent attacks of asthma, worse at night, and especially after midnight. Chronic enlargement of glands of posterior wall of pharynx. Puffiness of face; prostration.

Euphrasia. "Irritation and sneezing all day, with copious, bland discharge from the nose; conjunctivitis, with acrid, excoriating discharge from the eyes; great photophobia, with constant tendency to blink."

Gelsemium. This remedy may be indicated during the early stage. Great physical weakness. Patient subject to neuralgia as a result of chronic rhinitis. Intense occipital or frontal headache. Violent sneezing, with tingling in the nose.

Ipecac. Frequent sneezing. Paroxysms of asthma, with large accumulation of mucus in the air passages; sense of constriction in the throat and chest; worse from motion.

Kali iod. Implication of the frontal sinuses and maxillary cavities; discharge watery, colorless and excoriating. Eustachian tubes are frequently involved. Throbbing and burning pains in nasal and frontal bones. Aggravation latter part of the day and at night; nightly asthmatic attacks. With this remedy my best results have been with the 1x or 2x trituration, or in a saturated solution. More palliative than curative.

Sabadilla. Great itching of the nasal membrane, with violent paroxysms of sneezing; profuse, watery discharge from nose and eyes; worse in open air and from exposure to bright sunlight. Dry, spasmodic cough.

Sanguinaria nit. For the June attacks. Fluent, excoriating discharge from nose; a burning, scalded and itching sensation in posterior nares and throat. Dry cough, worse at night; pain and pressure in upper part of the chest. Asthma.

Terpine hydrate has been highly recommended during the asthmatic attacks, in doses of fifteen minims, three times a day. Not more than sixty minims per day should be given.

Consult, also, *Artemisia*, *Euphorbia off.*, *Grindelia rob.*, *Hydrochloric acid*, *Nux vom.*, and *Sticta pulmon.*

Chapter X

NEUROSES OF THE NOSE

(ANOSMIA)

Etiology. Diminution, or loss of the sense of smell, is a frequent symptom in nasal diseases, especially of polypi, hypertrophic rhinitis and deflection of the septum. It frequently results from nasal stenoses, because the odorous particles floating in the atmosphere are prevented from coming in contact with the olfactory portion of the nostrils. It may also be occasioned by the destruction or impairment of the olfactory nerve terminals, the result of atrophic rhinitis. Anosmia often results from empyema of the ethmoid cells. Inhalation of acrid or pungent gases, and the use of snuffs containing astringents are likewise causes of this affection. Or it may be due to such intercranial lesions as hemorrhage of the anterior and middle meningeal sutures, tumors and syphilis, and impairment of the olfactory nerve in its continuity.

Symptoms. There exists a close connection between the sense of smell and the sense of taste. It has been demonstrated that the sense of taste consists in distinguishing, "the bitter, sweet, salt and acid qualities of substances brought in contact with the mucous membrane of the tongue and palate, and that the more delicate elements of the sense of taste are due entirely to the appreciation of their odor by the olfactory nerve."

The loss of the sense of smell may be unilateral or bilateral. The olfactory perception of the two nostrils should be tested separately. For this purpose the fragrant odors should be used, care being taken to occlude completely the nostril not being tested.

Prognosis. When anosmia depends on local causes relief may result from the removal of such causes, but where the sense of smell has been absent for from five to eight years a cure is somewhat improbable.

In congenital anosmia, also, where it is the result of brain lesion, the prognosis is decidedly unfavorable. When syphilis is the cause relief is frequently obtained by proper specific treatment.

Treatment. The treatment consists in the proper removal of all inter-nasal lesions demanding mechanical or surgical treatment.

Insufflation of sulphate of strychnia, one-thirtieth of a grain, is recommended.

The constant or interrupted electric current has been suggested, but is rarely beneficial.

The following remedies may be consulted: *Sanguinaria*, *Ammonium mur.*, *Kali nit.*, *Naturm mur.*, *Pulsatilla*, and *Sticta pul.*

HYPEROSMIA

Over-sensitiveness of olfaction is usually met with in hysteria and neurasthenia; and may be the result of lowered physical vitality.

In this condition an odor may be perceived for hours or days after its removal. When this is the case the patient may again be made to experience the odor by mental suggestion.

The sense of smell is occasionally over-acute during the monthly period.

In the uncivilized, dark-skinned races, and in many

of the lower animals, the sense of olfaction is markedly developed.

PAROSMIA

Parosmia or parosphresia is a condition in which there is a perversion of the sense of smell. Usually the illusion is of a disagreeable character.

The cause may be due to some brain lesion. The aura of an epileptic fit is frequently preceded by delusions of smell.

Parosmia is also met with in the insane, and in persons of marked neurotic temperament.

It may occur in lead-poisoning and in locomotor ataxia.

The prognosis and treatment of these neuroses must depend upon the cause.

Internally, the following remedies are suggested: *Asafœtida*, *Aurum*, *Calcarea carb.*, *Graphites*, *Ignatia*, the *Kalis*, *Nux moschata* and *Psorinum.*

ANÆSTHESIA

This affection of the nose is quite rare. It is due to paralysis of the fifth nerve, caused by tumors, syphilis, involving the brain and nasal mucosæ.

It may be present in severe hysterical attacks.

Anæsthesia of the nasal mucous membrane is usually associated with absence of the sense of taste.

Tickling the nasal mucous membrane will ordinarily prove effective in malingerers simulating unconsciousness.

NEURALGIA

Neuralgia of the nasal branches of the trigeminus is

occasionally seen. It may be due to hypertrophy of the turbinals, especially when the middle turbinal presses on the septum.

Neuralgia in the nostrils is sometimes associated with empyema of the maxillary cavity. It may be reflex from dental irritation, or acute otitis.

Treatment. In addition to removal of local hypertrophies, and the relief of other extraneous conditions, the treatment consists in mild alkaline solutions applied to the nostrils.

Cocaine or morphine solutions may be used. Five grains of common table salt finely triturated, and insufflated, it is claimed, quickly relieve the suffering.

Internally, *Aconite*, *Colocynth* and *Gelsemium*, are to be thought of.

REFLEX NASAL NEUROSES

During the past few years the term reflex irritation has served to cover a multitude of sensations that could not otherwise be accounted for. This has been the case especially when considering the diseases of the external orifices.

The nostrils in common with the other outlets of the body have received their share of attention.

Enthusiasm in special departments of medicine is to be commended, but it should not be carried to such an extent as to make the specialist's chosen field the centre around which the rest of the body is dependent.

In many cases of so-called reflex irritation the connection between the nose, as a causative factor, and the irritation experienced, is not always trustworthy, yet it has been demonstrated that abnormal conditions in the nose are reflected, or by the patient referred to other parts of the body.

As certain conditions of the genitalia, or digestive organs, aggravate and not infrequently cause nasal irritation, so the converse may sometimes be true, and phenomena experienced in other parts of the body may result from nasal abnormalities.

Nasal cough is quite common, as the result of the turbinals pressing against the septum; or hypertrophy of the floor of the nostril may also produce it. The patient always refers the irritation to the larynx. The cough occurs in violent paroxysms and is usually characterized by a short, hard barking, or metallic-like sound. It is more frequent during the day. Expectoration is absent, but there may be a slight discharge of saliva, which the patient will claim comes from the throat. The cough is preceded by dryness, or a tickling, or pricking sensation in the larynx; this irritation is usually confined to a small spot.

Redness of the end of the nose may be due to hypertrophic rhinitis; especially when the hypertrophy is more pronounced in the anterior part of the nostrils.

Tinnitus, pain in the ear, and itching of the external auditory canal, is sometimes due to nasal hypertrophy, or to a spur impinging on the opposite wall.

When using an aural speculum, cough referred to the larynx is common.

Headache, ocular affections and asthma depending on nasal disease, have been referred to in previous articles.

The profession is indebted to J. Noland Mackenzie

for exhaustive investigation along the line of reflex nasal neuroses.

Treatment. As in all forms of neuroses, it is essential that the constitutional condition by improved by attention to proper diet and exercise, and the use of all means to improve the patient's general health.

This class of cases will frequently tax the physician's ability to diagnose and locate the seat of irritation. But patience and careful examination will usually disclose the cause.

Chapter XI

EMPYEMA OF THE ACCESSORY CAVITIES

(MAXILLARY SINUS)

Etiology. Empyema of the antrum may be caused by the root of a bicuspid, or first molar tooth, entering the cavity, especially if the tooth be carious; by hypertrophic rhinitis or nasal polypi occluding the *ostium maxillare*, thus preventing proper æration of the cavity. The latter cause may give rise to an exaggerated secretion of the antrum with resulting inflammation and suppuration. Empyema may also result from erysipelas.

I have been consulted in cases where the empyema was directly traceable to exposure to intense cold. In one case there was absence of rhinitis, the sinus alone being attacked. Another unique case occurring in my practice, was due to the patient passing a fine blade of hay through the canal of the tooth into the cavity. After a long period of systemic treatment, improvement being slight, the tooth was extracted. The stem of hay was found in the tooth, having penetrated one-third of an inch into the antral cavity.

A case due to phosphorus poisoning, caused by the habit of chewing matches, is at present under my care.

I believe that facial neuralgia and recurring paroxysms of pain in the face, and anterior part of the head, are frequently due to diseased conditions of the accessory sinuses, especially when the pain is followed by thin creamy, or yellowish discharge from one nostril.

Symptoms. Pain of an intermitting character is usually present, this may become so intense as to be almost unbearable. I have frequently noticed that the pain comes and stops suddenly. It is not gradual in its onset, but attacks instantly, then after remaining a few seconds, it as quickly ceases. During these paroxysms the face is often very red.

The pain extends to the brow and often to the ear on the affected side. The upper teeth feel elongated and are sensitive to a gentle tapping. The face is sensitive to pressure, especially at the points where the nerves

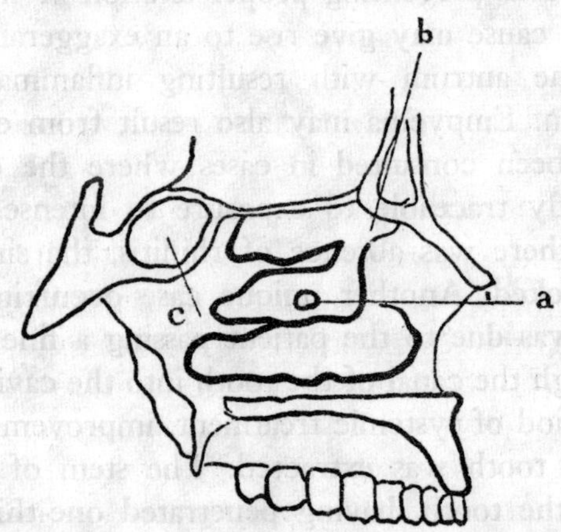

Fig. IX

emerge from the bony foramina. Swelling of the gum and inside of the cheek is frequent; the roof of the mouth, on the affected side, may also present a boggy and somewhat mottled appearance.

When the purulent collection is retained in the cavity for years, it not infrequently causes caries of the maxillary bone, and burrows through the outer wall of the alveolus into the mouth.

Diagnosis. During the past few years antral disease has been encountered more often than formerly. This is probably the result of the influenza epidemic, which in many cases produced nasal and throat inflammation. Because of the greater attention given to these conditions, and to the improved methods of examination, the diagnosis is not as difficult as formerly.

Frequently the history of the case will aid in arriving at a diagnosis. When a decayed bicuspid or molar tooth is at fault it may be found sensitive to pressure. Not infrequently there will be a history of alveolar abscess in the region of the affected tooth; or the stump may be filled, or "capped," thus preventing drainage and resulting in abscess. If the patient lies upon the healthy side the pus may enter the upper nostril. After reducing the lower and middle turbinal with cocaine and instructing the patient to lean forward and place his head between his knees, pus will be seen, on raising the head, between the lower and middle turbinals.

Transillumination affords exceptional value in establishing a diagnosis. To accomplish this I use a rubber cloth, placed over the patient's head and my own, in such a way as totally to exclude the light. An electric lamp–six to eight volts–is placed in the patient's mouth. Turning on the current, opacity will be observed on the diseased side toward the orbital notch, or it may correspond to the floor of the cavity. By making frequent interruptions of the light the patient perceives slight flashes in the eye on the sound side. On the diseased side the subjective flashes are less distinct or may be absent.

Using a curved syringe to inject hydrogen peroxide

into the cavity, through the nasal opening (Fig. IX, *a.*), is advocated. In many cases this is practicable, while in others it is extremely difficult to pass the point of the syringe into the *osteum.*

Aspirating the cavity, through the lower meatus, is another method of diagnosis; this is not commended, as the aspirating tube may fail to withdraw contained pus. Of the various exploratory openings, the one over the canine fossa is the best. This is made by dissecting up a small piece of the membrane, then passing a trephine, or drill, backwards, slightly inward, and in a horizontal direction until the cavity is entered. In this location food is not liable to enter the antrum.

Puncturing or drilling through the cavity of an extracted tooth, or through the alveolar process over the bicuspid, or first molar, may be advisable.

An opening through one of these places will enter the floor of the antrum, thus reaching the pyogenic cavity in its lowest part.

After making an exploratory opening into the antrum from the lower meatus, the socket of a tooth, or through the alveolus, an injection of hydrogen peroxide into the cavity will be followed when pus is present by the characteristic foam.

This is pathognomonic of antral empyema.

Prognosis. When the result of acute rhinitis, resolution follows the subsidence of the acute condition.

Cases of long standing, the result of chronic rhinitis, polypi, erysipelas, traumatism, or phosphorus poisoning, may be rebellious, requiring prolonged treatment to effect a cure.

Treatment. The treatment is both medical and surgical. When the condition occurs with nasal polypi, hypertrophic rhinitis, or empyema of the ethmoid and frontal sinuses, these conditions must first be relieved.

For the purpose of local treatment to the cavity, applications through its natural outlet into the nostril is to be preferred.

When this method fails to give satisfactory results, an opening must be made into the cavity through the alveolus. For this purpose a drill, or trephine (not less than one-eighth inch in diameter) is to be used.

To prevent the closing of the artificial entrance a drainage tube is necessary. This may be hard rubber, silver or gold. Myles' tubes are especally constructed for this purpose.

Various solutions are used for cleansing the cavity. Care must be taken in cleaning not to use great force, as the pressure of the liquid on the antral wall is liable to perpetuate the inflammatory condition. No one solution is applicable to all cases, and, in fact, each case may require frequent changing of the lotion.

Injections can be accomplished by means of a small piston syringe, to the end of which is attached a soft rubber tube; or the bulb syringe will answer.

Peroxide of hydrogen must not be continued for a prolonged period, as its constant use is too irritating.

The solutions to be preferred are: boracic acid, pyoktanin, sulpho-carbolate of zinc, resorcin, carbolic acid, permanganate of potash, and biniodide of mercury.

Occasionally it is necessary to use dry dressings, as iodol, aristol, boracic acid, or even one of the many preparations on the market containing iodine in various combinations. In rebellious cases it may be necessary to enlarge the opening above the alveolus, curette the cavity, and pack with gauze.

Curetting is apt to be accompanied by profuse hemorrhage, but the bleeding is quickly controlled by the gauze packing.

Decided swelling of the face and neck always occurs after the latter operation, but it usually subsides within three or four days.

FRONTAL SINUSES

Etiology. Empyema of the frontal sinuses may be due to blocking of their outlets by polypi, hypertrophy of the nasal membrane, or enlargement of the superior or middle turbinal. The more common causes are traumatism, syphilis, and disease of the ethmoid cells.

In nearly all cases of acute rhinitis, the frontal sinuses partake of the catarrhal inflammation, but it subsides with the acute nasal congestion.

Symptoms. There is present a sense of fulness, and headache above the nose and brow. As the secretions accumulate the distress may become intense. Paroxysms of shooting pain are frequent. Externally the frontal region is sensitive to contact.

When the accumulation discharges into the nostril, the pain quickly subsides, but in many cases recurs within a few days. This condition continues from the fall to the spring months, followed by relief during the summer, only to recur on the advent of cold weather.

The purulent product may accumulate until it causes displacement of the eyeball and decided œdema of the surrounding tissue. Or the orbital plate may be partially destroyed, permitting the escape of pus, and an abscess form in the orbital cavity.

In the same way erosion of the posterior wall may occur, the pus escaping into the brain cavity, with consequent meningitis.

Diagnosis. The history of the case, and location of pain with tenderness on pressure, will usually indicate disease of the frontal sinuses.

Prognosis. When the disease has existed for some time, a cure can be accomplished only by making an opening into the cells, destroying the pyogenic membrane, and re-opening the natural passages into the nostrils.

Treatment. A four per cent. solution of cocaine thoroughly applied to the upper part of the nostrils, with an atomizer, will frequently reduce the turgescence sufficiently to permit the retained secretions to pass through the infundibulum, (Fig. IX, *b.*)

It may be possible to pass a probe through the nostrils into the frontal sinuses, but great care should be observed in order not to injure the mucous membrane.

Where an abscess of the orbital cavity exists it must be opened. A probe can then be used to explore for necrosed bone. When it becomes imperative to open the frontal sinuses from the outside, the line of incision should extend along the lower border of the supraorbital ridge. The bleeding may be quite free. After this is stopped the periosteum is to be separated and drawn upwards and downwards. The opening through the bone is to be made either with a gouge and mallet, or a trephine. The opening must be large enough to permit of free inspection. The lining walls are to be thoroughly scraped with a curette, for the purpose of destroying the pyogenic membrane and granulations which are present.

A probe is then passed from the sinus into the nostril, after which a drainage tube is inserted, the lower extremity of which projects from the anterior nares.

Through the drainage tube irrigation must be used once or twice a day. The external wound is to be plugged with antiseptic gauze and dressings of the same kind applied.

This cannot be too strongly insisted upon, as erysipelas shows a predilection for this locality.

SPHENOID SINUSES

Etiology. The cause of catarrhal inflammation and empyema in the sphenoid sinuses, is much the same as in the other accessory cavities. Purulent accumulations have been noted after cerebro-spinal meningitis, erysipelas and typhoid fever. Or it may be due to an extension of inflammation from the posterior ethmoid cells.

Symptoms. The pain is deep-seated, and the patient refers the weight and pain to the middle region of the head. Mucus or pus is discharged into the post-nasal space. The secretion may be muco-purulent, or thin and purulent. When the bone is diseased the discharge is of a caseous consistency.

The various branches of the trifacial nerve may be involved.

Sudden blindness may occur, due to pressure on the optic nerve. When such is the case, an ophthalmoscope examination will show swelling of the optic disk.

Diagnosis. From the peculiar position of these cavities,

an exact diagnosis is often attended with considerable difficulty. Deep-seated pain in the head, bright yellow pus in the upper part of the nostril between the middle turbinal and the septum, sudden amaurosis, and pus on the posterior end of the superior turbinal, will render the diagnosis certain.

Prognosis. In chronic cases the prognosis must be guarded. Owing to the proximity of the sphenoidal sinus to the brain, an extension of the inflammation and necrosis of the sphenoid bone may result.

Treatment. Alkaline sprays and douches for cleansing the parts should be used. When nasal polypi, or hypertrophies are present, they should be removed as directed under previous chapters.

Pus in the sphenoid cavities is to be treated on the same principle as pus occurring elsewhere, *i.e.*, measures should be taken to evacuate it.

There are two methods proposed for entering the cavity.

The first is through the anterior nares by means of a narrow sharp gouge. The instrument is carried along the upper border of the middle turbinal, to about the junction of its middle and posterior thirds. The gouge is then passed upward and backward, when it can be made to penetrate the cavity at its lowest part. Or a nasal trephine propelled by an electric motor can be substituted for the gouge and with additional safety. (Fig. IX, *c*.)

After an opening has been made into the cavity, by either of these instruments, a curette should be used to remove the retained secretion and carious bone.

In the second method, the under wall of the cavity

is punctured through the vault of the pharynx.

The after treatment is of importance, and consists in the daily douching of the cavity with alkaline solutions, followed by antiseptic washes.

ETHMOID CELLS

Etiology. Empyema of the ethmoid cells is usually produced by hypertrophic rhinitis, or polypi, blocking the *ostium ethmoidale*.

It may be the result of facial erysipelas, scrofula or syphilis. Or it may extend from the neighboring cavities.

Symptoms. In purulent collections in the anterior ethmoid cells, many authors refer to pain as an invariable symptom. This I believe is a mistake, as pain is not usually pronounced unless the posterior ethmoid and the sphenoid cells are involved.

The middle turbinal is always enlarged, and usually presses on the septum. The turbinal is constantly bathed in a bright yellow pus, or the discharge may be of a light caseous character. During the early stage of the disease, the patient is aware of a fetid odor, but as the disease progresses the sense of smell is destroyed.

At times there may be a slight swelling of the external nose and the cheek of the affected side, with redness of the skin along the infra-orbital ridge.

Victims of this disease are often mentally depressed, and the general health suffers.

I have noticed in many of these cases a melancholic expression of the face. It is possible this may be due to the constant purulent discharge and attending fetor.

Diagnosis. Ordinarily, in uncomplicated cases, the diagnosis is not difficult. In many cases there is a similar condition in the antrum. However, in empyema of the maxillary cavity, the discharge is from the middle meatus; whereas in ethmoid disease the purulent secretion is in the middle meatus and also on the middle turbinal.

Polypi and granulations are frequent complications in ethmoidal disease. The middle turbinal bone is always soft, and breaks down under pressure of the probe. Bleeding is rare.

Prognosis. Suppurative disease of the ethmoid cells always runs a chronic course, extending over years and frequently exists for life.

There is a danger of the purulent condition extending to the orbital cavity and possibly to the brain.

Treatment. Nasal hypertrophies and polypi, when present, must first be removed. In many cases it becomes necessary to remove a portion of the middle turbinal bone. This is easily accomplished by curved scissors, cutting forceps, the snare, or the trephine. After a part of the turbinal is removed, the cells must then be curetted.

I have more than once been surprised at the great quantity of pus and *debris* removed. When a carious condition exists, and the intercellular walls are not already destroyed, they can be broken down.

The daily washing of the cavities by alkaline and antiseptic lotions should be continued until all purulent secretion has ceased to form.

Cocaine anæsthesia is usually sufficient in chronic cases, as the operation is not painful.

Ablation of the cap of the middle turbinal and curetting the ethmoid cells is not a bloody operation, as removal of carious bone in any part of the body is not attended by severe bleeding.

Coexisting empyema in the other cavities must be treated as suggested under their respective headings.

Therapeutics

Arsenicum alb. Swelling of the face; burning stinging pains, aggravated at night, better in the open air. Face has an anxious expression.

Aurum met. Scrofula and syphilitico-mercurial cases. Drawing, tearing in left side of face; teeth feel too long; the bones of the head are exceedingly sensitive to pressure.

Chelidonium. "Right cheek bones feel as if swollen, violent tearing in maxillary antrum."

Cinchona. Neuralgia, periodical attacks, skin sensitive to least touch; or exposure to cold air. Pains mostly infra-orbital and maxillary branches.

Fluoric acid. Nightly bone pains, the result of syphilis or abuse of mercury.

Hepar sulphur. Bones of the face painful to touch; headache at root of nose; throbbing pains.

Kali hydriodicum. The result of syphilis. Fulness and tightness at root of nose, with beating in nasal bones; darting pain extending to the ear. Pains worse at night.

Phosphorus. Twitching, darting and tension in cheek bones; burning and throbbing in region of antrum.

Silicea. Ulceration from phosphorus poisoning, with discharge thin and watery. Fistulous openings hard to heal.

Staphisagria. Inflammation of the bones of the face; darting pain in the antrum.

The following remedies may also be consulted: *Hecla lava*, *Kalmia*, *Magnesium phos.*, *Mercurius*, *Nitric acid*, and *Spigelia*.

Chapter XII

ACUTE PHARYNGITIS

Synonyms. Acute inflammation of the pharynx. Acute sore throat. Ulcerated sore throat. Angina faucium.

Definition. Acute pharyngitis is an acute inflammation of the pharynx, frequently implicating the larynx, and nostrils.

Etiology. Idiopathic. One of the most common causes, is the condition commonly called "catching cold." Exposure to sudden changes in temperature, as going from a hot room into the cold air, living in badly ventilated and over-heated rooms, sitting in a draught, or a sudden chilling after violent exercise.

It may be the result of repelled cutaneous eruptions, or may be reflex from genito-urinary and gastro-intestinal derangements, especially in those prone to constipation.

The condition is frequent in children when the upper part of the body is over-clothed. This causes the child to perspire, and renders it more susceptible to changes in the atmosphere. During certain seasons pharyngitis is highly epidemic and contagious.

Recent investigation has shown that the staphylococci and streptococci which are normally present in the healthy mouth are greatly increased in number during damp and cold weather, and may excite pharyngitis.

It has been noticed that influenza-epidemics in horses are frequently followed by similar conditions in the human family, with complicating pharyngitis.

The *traumatic* form is due to swallowing hot liquids, inhaling steam, or acrid vapors; or it may be caused by fish-bones injuring the membranes. Irritating food may also cause it.

Follicular. In this form of acute pharyngitis the follicles on the posterior wall are principally involved, although the surrounding tissue is implicated. The inflammation of the glands is more pronounced in this form of the disease.

Septic. Frequently called ulcerated sore throat, or hospital sore throat. This condition is often seen in first-year medical students who spend much of their time in the dissecting room. It was formerly of frequent occurrence in hospital nurses, but since more attention has been given to asepsis and cleanliness, it is rarely met in hospitals.

Exposure to vitiated air, as sewer-gas or decaying organic matter, may give rise to septic pharyngitis.

It may also be caused by drinking impure water.

Symptoms. The character and severity of the symptoms will depend on the cause and nature of the attack. In mild cases the throat feels dry; there is pain on speaking or swallowing, which frequently extends to the ear.

Severer attacks may be preceded by a chill, or chilly sensation, headache, languor, sense of constriction or tightness of the throat, severe pain on swallowing, etc. There is present a short, dry cough and an almost constant desire to hawk or clear the throat; though for the first few days there is little or no secretion. Later there is a mucous discharge which gradually changes to a muco-pus.

In the epidemic form small, yellowish patches are common on the pharynx and tonsils.

Some degree of rhinitis or laryngitis is always present; when inflammatory condition extends downward hoarseness is present.

The palate, uvula and tonsils frequently partake of the inflammation. The tongue is heavily coated and attended by a bad taste.

The fever may be high; in severe septic cases it is not unusual for the thermometer to register 104°F.

An examination reveals dilated blood vessels and a reddened condition of the pharynx. In severe cases the mucous membrane of the tonsils and uvula are inflamed, and, in addition, there may be œdema of the uvula and arches of the palate. The glands on the wall of the pharynx are frequently enlarged to the size of a split pea.

When the condition is the result of traumatism, œdema of the pharynx and larynx may be so great as to cause asphyxia, necessitating tracheotomy.

The sub-lingual and cervical glands are often swollen. Turning the head and pressure on the neck are painful.

Diagnosis. Acute pharyngitis may be confounded with tonsillitis and diphtheria.

In *tonsillitis* the brunt of the attack is confined to the tonsils. The external glands are more enlarged while the anterior pillars are more inflamed.

Diphtheria is usually ushered in by nose-bleed and vomiting. During the first two days the temperature is not as high as in pharyngitis, and the membrane tends to spread. It is not in isolated spots as is the case in the milder disease.

It must not be forgotten that diphtheria may be engrafted on a simple sore throat.

Prognosis. In catarrhal cases the prognosis is always good. The disease lasts from three days to a week.

One attack predisposes to another, as frequently the parts are left in a susceptible condition. When caused by traumatism the prognosis will necessarily depend on the character and location of the injury.

Septic cases are often dangerous, as an abscess may form in the deeper tissues of the neck; or, as a sequel, paralysis of the soft palate may occur.

Treatment. The bowels should always be moved, preferably by enemata, or one of the bitter waters. Often the attack is preceded by constipation or digestive derangements. Local applications, by means of an atomizer, are usually beneficial.

Gargling, so generally recommended, is rarely advisable, for the reason that the solution does not reach the inflamed membrane; and, further, it increases the pain by bringing into action muscles that should be kept at rest.

During the early stage, when the mucous membrane is dry, astringents should not be applied. I cannot recommend steam inhalations, as I believe they prolong the attack, and, not infrequently, are followed by laryngeal and bronchial irritation.

Sometimes clothes wrung from hot or cold water and applied around the neck are grateful.

For spraying with the atomizer, one of the indicated internal remedies may be used in aqueous solution; or menthol, ten grains; cocaine, five grains, to water, one ounce, will aid in reducing the congestion and relieving pain. In the ulcerated form permanganate of potash, carbolic acid, peroxide of hydrogen, or one of the many antiseptic preparations of the market will be useful.

Therapeutics

Aconite. Early in the attack. High fever, dry skin, restless, excitable. Fauces dark red, burning. Pricking, burning, extending along eustachian tube; hoarseness. After sudden changes in temperature from warm to intense cold.

Ammonium carb. Septic sore throat. Tonsils bluish, covered with offensive mucus; tendency to ulceration; burning and roughness in the throat.

Apis. Tonsils and throat bright red, uvula and border of soft palate œdematous. Tenacious mucus in throat. Breathing and swallowing difficult; burning, stinging pains.

Baptisia. Septic sore throat. Fauces dark red. Ulcers on posterior wall and tonsils. Sense of constriction in throat; unusual absence of pain. Can swallow nothing but liquids.

Belladonna. Fauces and pharynx deep red, shining; sense of constriction in throat, painful swallowing, liquids are ejected through the nose. Fever, thirst, face hot and swollen, dilated pupils. Throbbing headache; the arterial action very decided.

Cantharis. Throat feels on fire and covered with vesicles, much swollen; swallowing of liquids difficult.

Chininum ars. Septic cases, great exhaustion. Bloody ulcers in the throat; uvula gangrenous; exudation on pharyngeal wall; swallowing of liquids very difficult.

Ferrum phos. Early in attack; throat red, spots of congestion, pain and throbbing. Uvula relaxed.

Kali nit. Burning, cutting pain; scraping in throat; uvula and tonsils red.

Mercurius. Painful dryness of the throat, mouth full of soliva; uvula swollen, stinging worse from empty swallowing, at night and in cold air. Glands swollen.

Nitric acid. Pricking as from a splinter in the throat, worse when swallowing. Sense of constriction in the pharynx, making swallowing difficult; stitches in throat.

Sanguinaria. Roof of mouth and uvula sore and burning. Throat feels swollen to suffocation, with pain when swallowing. Ulcerated sore throat. Throat so dry feels as though it would crack; better inhaling cold air.

Consult Therapeutics under Tonsillitis; also Acute Laryngitis.

HERPETIC PHARYNGITIS

Synonyms. Benign membranous sore throat. Aphthous sore throat. Cankered sore throat.

Etiology. This form of sore throat is more commonly seen in children, especially in those of a scrofulous nature, although it is not uncommon in adults. It usually develops during the changeable weather of the spring and fall months. Exposure to septic influences which implicates the throat, as imperfect house drainage, decaying vegetable mattter and septic diseases, are not infrequent causes. Mental emotions and menstrual irregularities are likewise noted by writers as causes. It may also result from neuropathic disturbances.

Symptoms. The condition is preceded, for a few days,

by malaise, drowsy condition, headache; and there may be slight chilliness; during this time gastric disturbance with loss of appetite is common. This is followed by fever, thirst and sore throat. The submaxillary glands are usually swollen.

Owing to absence of pain in the beginning, the symptoms may be misleading.

In the early stage the fauces are redder than normal. In two or three days there appear small vesicles on the pharyngeal wall and soft palate; these ruptures are replaced by a thin membranous exudation, often of a stringy character. Fever may be quite high and prostration pronounced.

Diagnosis. Membranous sore throat is frequently mistaken for diphtheria. There are cases in which the differential diagnosis is a difficult matter. I fully agree with Laird: "That remedies which have been employed more or less successfully in the former malady may thus acquire an unmerited reputation for efficacy in the treatment in the graver disease."

The exudation in the milder condition is in isolated patches scattered over the soft palate, tonsils and pharynx, and is sometimes found on the inside of the cheeks and gums. At times herpes of the anus and prepuce are present.

The exudation of herpes has not the compact buckskin appearance of diphtheria.

Prognosis. When uncomplicated the prognosis is good. In young children laryngeal œdema may result. During diphtheria epidemics the more serious disease may follow.

Treatment. Sprays containing hydrogen peroxide.

one part to water three parts; permanganate of potash five grains to water one ounce; and carbolic acid, five to ten drops to water one ounce, are useful.

At times it may be necessary to wipe off the exudation with a cotton-tipped applicator before applying the spray.

Therapeutics

Apis. Stinging pains, dryness, small gray ulcers in the throat, œdematous condition. Great prostration; urine highly colored.

Kali bich. Tough, stringy mucus in the throat; small patches on the tonsils. Ulcers in the fauces discharging cheesy lumps of offensive smell.

Mercurius proto. Patches of mucus on posterior wall, and small spots which look ulcerated. Tenacious mucus, fetid smell. Salivary glands swollen. Thick yellow coating on the tongue.

Kali chlor. White or grayish patches on throat; patches on inside of cheeks and gums.

Consult *Hepar sulph.*, *Lachesis* and *Natrum sulph.* (See articles on Acute Pharyngitis and Tonsillitis.)

RHEUMATIC PHARYNGITIS

Rheumatism of the pharynx is probably more common than is generally supposed. Many cases diagnosed as recurring acute pharyngitis, and exacerbations of chronic pharyngitis, are undoubtedly of a rheumatic character.

The condition may co-exist with rheumatism in other parts of the body, but it is more often confined to the pharyngeal region.

9

Lithæmia, and the uric acid diathesis, seem to favor it. Men are somewhat more subject to the affection than women.

Inspection may show a slight congestion of the fauces, or posterior wall. The patient complains of aching or stiffness in the pharynx and sometimes the same painful conditions are experienced in muscles of the neck. When the latter is the case, wry-neck may be present.

The pain is characterized by its sudden onset, disappearing as quickly as it came.

The treatment consists in attention to the general health and relief of any underlying dyscrasia.

In these cases, the free use of Fonticello Lithia Water is beneficial. Dry heat, such as bags of hot salt, or hot flannels, applied to the neck, will often modify the pain.

Therapeutics

Consult *Bryonia*, *Ferrum phos.*, *Guaiacum*, *Rhus tox.*, and *Salicylic acid.*

ERYSIPELAS OF THE PHARYNX

Etiology. The cause is probably the same as the cause of erysipelas in other parts of the body.

The disease may extend from the face to the pharynx; or, as is more frequently the case, it may develop primarily in the pharynx, and gradually extend to the larynx, or spread to the external integument.

Symptoms. When occurring primarily in the pharynx, it may be preceded for two or three days by headache, pain in the back, elevated temperature, and swelling of the cervical glands. Soon swallowing becomes painful, the throat is very hot, dry and glazed œdema of the pharyngeal mucosa, uvula and soft palate is frequent. At times blisters filled with serum or pus appear on the faucial wall; when these break, ulceration and gangrene may ensue. The tongue is thickly coated, soon becoming dry, dark-red cracks and small blackish crusts appear.

Diagnosis. When the disease appears first on the skin, the diagnosis is not difficult. But when occurring primarily in the throat, it may be impossible to diagnose the disease, for the first two or three days, or at least until the characteristic blisters appear.

Prognosis. In case of extreme debility and in alcoholics, the result is apt to be fatal. In all cases the prognosis must be guarded, as œdema, dyspnœa and death by suffocation may quickly ensue.

Treatment. Local applications should be of a soothing character. A spray of menthol, five to ten grains, to albolene, one ounce, is grateful. Peroxide or hydrogen, sucking ice and the use of morphine are not advisable. The use of the first named drug will increase the smarting, and the foam resulting after its use causes narrowing of the breathing space. Sucking ice may be grateful, for the time being, but its use is followed by greater dryness.

If œdema, threatening suffocation ensues, hypodermic injections of pilocarpine hydrochlorate, one-fourth grain, may be used; or scarification of the œdematous tissues may be necessary. If all other measures fail to relieve, tracheotomy must be performed.

Owing to the high fever and severe pain in swallowing, debility quickly ensues. Nutritious semi-solid food should be given; when pain, on swallowing becomes severe, nutrient enemata must be given.

Therapeutics

Apis. This remedy is the similimum in, perhaps, the majority of cases. The main indications are œdema, burning, stinging pains, bright redness of the mucous membrane, small blisters on the back part of the throat.

Arsenicum alb. Burning and dryness in fauces. Great prostration; the patient is restless; the condition assumes a typhoid character. There is an absence of the great œdema and stinging pains indicating *Apis*.

Belladonna. Fauces and roof of mouth deep red; swallowing is painful; the throat feels constricted. Great arterial congestion; throbbing in head; face intensely flushed.

Rhus tox. External swelling; glands enlarged; cellular tissue of neck infiltrated.

Compare *Cantharis*, *Lachesis*, *Mercurius*, and *Muriatic acid*.

SIMPLE CHRONIC PHARYNGITIS

Synonyms. Chronic sore throat. Relaxed sore throat.

Etiology. In many cases simple chronic pharyngitis is the result of repeated attacks of acute pharyngitis, and acute rhinitis.

In all forms of rhinitis the pharynx is implicated to a greater or less extent. This cannot be otherwise, owing to the continuity of the nasal and pharyngeal mucous membranes. A blocking of the nostrils with an increase of their normal secretions passing backwards, and the resulting mouth breathing permits the outer air with its attending impurities to come directly in contact with the pharynx. This must necessarily cause an inflamed condition of the mucous membrane and glands of the pharyngeal wall.

The use of alcoholic liquors, and excessive smoking, will also cause or aggravate the condition.

In addition, disorders of the digestive organs, and in women uterine diseases are a frequent cause of chronic pharyngitis.

Straining the voice, as in shouting, is a frequent cause in young men.

Symptoms. The patient complains that in the morning there is dried mucus in the throat, which requires considerable effort to remove it. The throat feels dry and parched, and hemming and hawking are frequent, which may be followed by slight mucous expectoration.

The voice is usually weak and soon tires when speaking. Various other sensations, as a feeling of constriction in the throat, and localized pricking and smarting may be complained of. A tickling cough is frequent; this may be due to adhesive mucus, or to elongation of the uvula. Inspection shows the posterior wall to be congested, not uniformly, but in patches; the blood vessels are enlarged and full. The lateral walls of the pharynx back of the posterior pillars, usually present a vertical strip of reddened and enlarged tissue. When this is present, tinnitus and pain in the ears are frequent, which is more noticeable in changeable weather.

Prognosis. The result depends upon the exciting cause. In nearly all cases the patient should be given to understand that prolonged treatment is necessary. In this condition, patience on the part of both the physician and patient, must be exercised, Gradual improvement is the rule.

Treatment. In all cases the primary cause must be sought for, and treatment directed to the removal of such cause.

Constipation and hepatic, digestive and uterine disorders must be corrected. Hypertrophic rhinitis, when present, should be first reduced. Locally, tenacious or adhering mucus must be removed, either by mild alkaline sprays or by a cotton-wrapped applicator.

Soothing sprays are usually grateful to the patient, and their use is rarely contra-indicated. The atomizer should be provided with a curved tip. This is passed through the mouth and directed behind and above the border of the soft palate. When in place the patient closes his lips on the tube and breathes through the nose. A few quick compressions of the rubber bulb will serve to throw the spray on the vault and walls of the pharynx. Patients frequently complain that they cannot use the post-nasal spray satisfactorily. With the aid of a mirror, to enable the patient to properly place the tip, it is ordinarily an easy matter to spray the post-nasal space.

The following remedies in aqueous solution have been recommended as useful for spraying: copper sulphate, ten grains to the ounce; alum fifteen to twenty-five grains to the ounce; sulphate of zinc, ten grains to the ounce; hamamelis, one part to four parts of water, is useful when the venous blood vessels are prominent. Bichloride of mercury, one-fourth grain to the ounce of albolene will frequently give good results. Oily sprays are to be preferred to the aqueous, for the reason that the oil remains longer on the membrane.

Nitrate of silver, twenty to thirty grains to the ounce of water, is an excellent local application in chronic pharyngitis. A small piece of cotton is tightly wrapped on a curved applicator, dipped in the silver solution, the superfluous liquid pressed out by blotting paper, or between the stopper and neck of the bottle. This may be applied once every three or four days. Because the use of the nitrate of silver has been abused when applied to mucous surfaces should not prevent the use of so valuable an agent when properly applied.

Therapeutics

(See Chronic Follicular Pharyngitis.)

CHRONIC FOLLICULAR PHARYNGITIS

Etiology. This form of pharyngitis, commonly called clergyman's sore throat, is so named because the condition is frequent in ministers and public speakers, who are required to make special use of their voice. Yet it must not be inferred that the condition is found only in that class. An ordinary conversational tone with faulty method of voice production may produce it.

The various causes and symptoms given in the previous article (simple chronic pharyngitis) will also apply to this condition. In addition, I believe one of the greatest causes in producing faulty or "throaty voice" is a lack of proper instruction in colleges and seminaries as to the proper method of using the voice for public speaking.

Lowering the voice to a whisper, then suddenly

raising it to its extreme limit, must necessarily cause congestion of the mucous membrane. And the unnatural guttural tones which are supposed to be impressive cannot be too strongly condemned.

Symptoms. In the follicular form of pharyngitis the posterior pharyngeal wall is seen dotted with small, reddish elevations; these are the enlarged follicles. They exude a viscid secretion, which at times is of a cheesy character.

I cannot agree with the opinion expressed in many of the special works devoted to laryngology, that the fetid odor, so frequently complained of, is caused by the follicular exudation. In my opinion the fetor is usually due to the tonsillar exudation.

When the glands on the vault of the pharynx are involved, or, when they are enlarged as the result of adenoid hypertrophy, the secretion is of a greenish color, and is difficult of removal. As a result of hypertrophy in the upper part of the pharynx, deafness is frequent.

Hawking and repeated efforts to clear the throat are more frequent than in the simple catarrhal form. Huskiness is common and is due to implication of the larynx.

Prognosis. In nearly all cases the condition can be cured, or greatly relieved. But in the case of public speakers, when the trouble has existed for a long time, the voice may be so weakened that further public speaking is impossible.

Treatment. In professional voice-users the first thing to insist on is a proper use of the voice. So long as the vocal organs are improperly used a cure of all the abnormal pharyngeal conditions is impossible. The surgeon might as well expect a perfect result in a broken arm, when the patient constantly uses it, as to look for a cure in chronic pharyngitis, or chronic laryngitis, when faulty voice production is continued.

When exudation is present it should be removed by gently pressing the glands with forceps. The cheesy matter will be expelled as a little hard lump, or it may present the appearance of a small worm.

It is often advisable to destroy the larger follicles; for this purpose the galvano-cautery is to be preferred; in the absence of a proper battery the milder acids, as glacial acetic, or trichlor-acetic, may be used, but care must be exercised not to burn the surrounding tissues.

In using the galvano-cautery the platinum should be in small straight wires, or, preferably, in cork-screw shape. It is often necessary to destroy the larger blood vessels; this is best accomplished by making one or two punctures in each vessel with the galvano-cautery point.

But no application of a destructive character is to be applied to the throat except when the parts are brought into view with a strong light.

Local applications, in the form of sprays, are frequently required. Those suggested under Simple Chronic Pharyngitis may be used. The main requirement is to have the solution an astringent. As new remedies are placed on the market every few weeks a more extended list of drugs for spraying is not necessary.

Therapeutics

Æsculus hip. Ropy mucus of a sweetish taste; fauces dark and congested; worse on left side. If portal congestion and the characteristic hæmorrhoidal symptoms are present this remedy may be given with assurance of relief.

Ammonium carb. Dry cough at night, as from dust. Pain in throat, as if right tonsil was swollen when swallowing. Sense of scraping in the throat down the œsophagus.

Antimonium crud. Thick, yellowish mucus in posterior nares; rawness of the palate. Tongue coated thick, milky-white.

Argentum met. Viscid, gray, jelly-like mucus in the throat. Throat feels raw and sore during expiration, swallowing or coughing. "Expectoration of lumps of pure mucus, like boiled starch."

Arsenicum iod. Enlarged follicles on posterior wall of pharynx, with burning and rawness. Tonsils enlarged. In morning hawks up thick mucus mixed with blood. Mucous membrane anæmic, with interlacing of small injected blood vessels. Adapted to the tuberculous and strumous diathesis.

Calcarea carb. When swallowing, feeling as if throat was too narrow. "Enlarged veins on soft palate and pharynx, giving rise to a bluish tinge. Thick, jelly-like, tough discharge." Scrofulous diathesis; the constitutional indications are often more pronounced than the local.

Calcarea phos. Hypertrophy of the pharyngeal follicles. Mucous membrane thickened. When first swallowing, dryness and burning. "On empty deglutition sensation of having swallowed uvula." Discharge yellowish-white, thick.

Capsicum. Uvula elongated. Mucous membrane dark red. Burning sensation in the throat. Ten drops of the tincture to two ounces of water, as a gargle, will often benefit.

Graphites. Palate feels sore, fauces reddened. Sensation of lump in the throat, especially at night. "Red, inflamed, scurfy, cracked, eczematous condition of mucous membrane." Hawking of offensive mucus.

Hamamelis. Stinging in uvula. Varicose condition of the blood vessels. When eating must drink large quantities of water to assist in swallowing.

Hepar sulph. Stitches in throat, extending to the ear. Sensation of splinter in the throat. Scraping in throat when swallowing. Uvula relaxed; follicles enlarged. Constant desire to hawk up mucus.

Hydrastis. Yellow, tenacious mucus in posterior nares; post-nasal dropping. Discharge is thick, yellow or greenish and fetid. Follicles enlarged. Aggravation from exposure to cold. Locally, one-half grain of the muriate to water one ounce.

Kali bich. Hawking of thick, tenacious mucus in the morning. Uvula relaxed. Sensation of plug in throat. Ulcers in the fauces, discharging cheesy lumps of offensive smell. Posterior wall of pharynx dark red. Follicles enlarged.

Kali mur. Mucous membrane pale and thin in patches. Stoppage of the eustachian tubes, deafness and adhesions of the drum-head.

Magnesium phos. Thickening of the posterior wall. Spasmodic cough.

Mercurius dulc. Mucous membrane dark red; dry, sore sensation; eustachian tubes involved. But the tongue is moist and covered with a whitish, thick coat. Breath fetid.

Nux vom. Throat feels sore, rough, as if scraped, especially when swallowing and inhaling cold air. Stitches in the ear when swallowing. Characteristic gastric symptoms.

Phosphorus. Rawness, dryness and scraping in the throat. Sensation of cotton in the throat.

Phytolacca. Fauces congested, dark red; dryness of the throat. Frequent desire to clear the throat.

Pulsatilla. Veins enlarged; mucous membrane bluish-red. Mouth dry, without thirst. Menstrual derangements cause asthmatic disturbances.

Rumex. Excoriated feeling in throat; secretion of mucus in posterior nares. Sensation of lump in the throat.

Sanguinaria. Roof of mouth sore and burning; heat in throat, better inhaling cold air. Throat feels dry, as if it would crack.

ATROPHIC PHARYNGITIS

Synonyms. Dry pharyngitis. Pharyngitis sicca.

Etiology. Atrophic pharyngitis is usually associated with atrophic rhinitis. It may also follow follicular pharyngitis; it not infrequently appears about the age of puberty, especially when adenoid tissue is present. Debility with anæmia seems to favor it.

Atrophic pharyngitis has frequently been noticed in Bright's disease and diabetes.

Symptoms. The most frequent complaint is dryness in the throat. This is due to failure of the glands and follicles to secrete and expel their normal mucus which is required to keep the parts moist. Sense of constriction in the throat and delay in swallowing are frequent; the latter is relieved after a few swallows of liquid.

Hawking, with a desire to clear the throat, is a common symptom. Inspection reveals the membrane dry and glazed, and often dry mucus is seen adhering to the wall. The outline of the cervical vertebræ can frequently be seen, especially in anæmic cases, and in old persons. At times the membrane may be decidedly paler than normal; or, the paleness may appear in patches only. The eustachian tubes frequently partake of the atrophic condition. Aural inspection will show calcareous deposits on the tympanum. Thickening takes place between the ossicles and walls of the cavity, resulting in tinnitus and deafness.

Prognosis. In young people the condition can generally be cured; but when deafness is pronounced, and in the aged, slight relief is all that can be expected.

Treatment. The nostrils and pharynx should be kept free from all adhering crusts. For this purpose an alkaline douche is best. After the parts are cleansed, a solution of nitrate of silver, five to ten grains to the ounce of water, applied by means of a cotton-wrapped applicator, will serve to stimulate the glands to renewed activity. Muriate of ammonia tablets, two grains each, are often useful, as the effect of this remedy is to moisten the pharyngeal membrane.

Swabbing with iodine and iodide of potash dissolved in glycerine, is often recommended. But in my hands it has frequently proved a failure. Galvanism has been used with benefit, the positive pole being placed to the pharynx. For the first two or three weeks, daily applications are necessary; after this period the current may be applied once or twice a week. Massage applied directly to the pharyngeal membrane by means of special instruments is highly recommended.

In this condition I cannot too strongly emphasize the necessity of constitutional treatment.

Change of climate will sometimes be followed by marked improvement in both the general health and in the atrophic condition.

THERAPEUTICS

Æsculus hip. Dry burning and constriction in fauces; frequent inclination to swallow.

Alumina. Great dryness, which induces frequent clearing of throat; sensation of a splinter in throat; rough voice; scraping sensation in naso-pharynx.

Cistus. Fauces very dry without feeling dry; at night must swallow saliva to relieve the sense of dryness; cold air causes pain in the throat.

Coccus cact. "Throat symptoms worse from warmth, especially at night;" burning and dryness in throat.

Hydrastis. Mucous membrane dry and glazed; throat feels sore and excoriated.

Kali bich. Dryness and soreness of soft palate; mucous membrane coppery; sense of constriction in throat; thick viscid mucus, difficult to remove from throat; cracking sensation in eustachian tubes and ears at night.

Sabadilla. Fauces dry, cannot swallow saliva on account of pain.

(Consult Atrophic Rhinitis; also Chronic Pharyngitis.)

PHARYNGO-MYCOSIS

Etiology. The etiology of the pharyngo-mycosis is

unknown. Formerly the condition was considered extremely rare. But during the past few years numerous cases have been reported in the medical journals. The favorite seat of the fungus is a hypertrophied tonsil; next in order the base of the tongue and the lateral pillars.

They appear as white or light yellowish projections, somewhat resembling an elongated wart, and rarely extend more than one-eighth of an inch above the surface.

Symptoms. There usually is a sense of fulness or obstruction in the throat. The fungus may produce tickling and smarting. A few cases are reported where the subjective symptoms were absent. When the growth occurs on the base of the tongue the use of a laryngeal mirror is required to bring it into view.

Prognosis. Although not dangerous, the condition is usually very stubborn in yielding to treatment.

Treatment. Local applications are wholly useless. The only successful treatment is to pull the fungus out with forceps, and then puncture the seat of the growth with the galvano-cautery. Or, puncture with the galvano-cautery alone will frequently answer.

The fungi are very tenacious. On attempting to pull them out with forceps they will stretch like a piece of rubber.

Chapter XIII

TUMORS OF THE PHARYNX

(BENIGN TUMORS)

Papillomata are the most common form of benign tumors of this region. They grow either from the uvula, tonsil or palate.

Symptoms. When small there are usually no subjective symptoms, but as the growth increases in size there are present the various symptoms incident to an obstruction. Pain is generally absent. The tumors vary in size from that of the head of a pain to a mass causing serious obstruction to respiration.

Papillomata are usually pedunculated and hang in clusters or, there may be one large tumor with a broad base. In a case on which I operated, a tumor, about the size of a small egg, was attached to the tonsil by a thick base. In all cases of pharyngeal tumors a microscopical examination will aid in arriving at a diagnosis. But entire dependence must not be placed on the microscope, unless there are other confirmatory symptoms.

Papillomatous growths occasionally recur after removal.

Treatment. The treatment consists in removing the tumor with the cold snare, cautery loop, or scissors.

The small, wart-like growths are best treated by daily applications of alcohol, or by destroying them with the galvano-cautery point.

MALIGNANT TUMORS

Round-cell sarcoma and epithelioma are the most

common forms of malignant tumors occurring in the pharynx.

Symptoms. Sarcoma is more likely to occur on the tonsil. It presents itself as a dark-red, round tumor with an even surface, which ulcerates as the disease progresses. It may occur at any period of life.

Epithelioma is paler, of a warty appearance, and ulceration is an early symptom. It generally appears after middle life.

Sarcoma in the pharynx is characterized by pain extending to the ear on swallowing, although this may not be severe until ulceration begins. As the growth increases, infiltration of the glands and surrounding tissues takes place. "On digital exploration the tumor gives the characteristic fixed indurated feeling of malignant tumors." (McBride.)

Emaciation is progressive; this is due to inability to eat, and also to the general septic condition.

Prognosis. If the case is seen before infiltration occurs in the surrounding tissue, an operation offers some hope of relief. But invariably the disease is fatal. Death from inanition, hæmorrhage or œdema of the larynx occurs in from three to twenty-four months.

Treatment. When the disease is confined to the tonsil, the gland may be enucleated through the mouth. Or, the growth may be removed by an external operation; this is often preferable, as it brings into view any enlarged cervical glands that are present, and permits their removal at the same operation. Before an external opening is made, a preliminary tracheotomy is advisable.

But usually the main indication is to relieve the

dysphagia and maintain the patient's strength.

(For further treatment and Therapeutics see Malignant Tumors of the Nose.)

FIBROMATA

Synonyms. Fibrous polypi.

Etiology. The immediate exciting cause of fibromata is not known. With few exceptions they have occurred in males between ten and thirty years of age. The tumor usually springs from the body of the sphenoid bone, the vomer, or the upper cervical vertebræ. A few cases are recorded where the point of attachment was on the lower turbinal.

Symptoms. One of the earliest symptoms is bleeding and nasal obstruction, with more or less muco-purulent discharge; or, it may be of a muco-sanguinolent character. At times the tumor may grow with wonderful rapidity, displacing cartilage and bone, and causing external deformity of the face. The nose becomes broadened and flattened, causing the so-called "frog-face." In other cases the growth may enter the nostril and extend toward the external opening. Or, it may extend downward in the pharynx and present below the border of the soft palate. The tumor is somewhat pedunculated, and the external surface is the color of the surrounding mucous membrane. Headache of a neuralgic character is frequently present. As the growth enlarges the eye may become involved and exophthalmus result.

Diagnosis. The location of the tumor, its tendency to bleed, and its dense character, usually render the diagnosis comparatively easy.

Prognosis. It is possible that spontaneous absorption may occur. But the tendency of the tumor is to become larger and to destroy the tissues with which it is in contact, causing necrosis and septicæmia. Or, sarcomatous degeneration may occur.

Treatment. The injection of acids and caustics into the tumor is to be avoided, as their use results in prolonged sloughing and tendency to septic infection. In a few cases electrolysis has proved a valuable aid. But usually extirpation by surgical means should be followed.

When the tumor is small, the galvano-cautery snare may be used. In larger growths, however, the larger-sized cold steel wire should be employed. The loop is made to encircle the tumor and is carried as close as possible to the point of attachment. The wire should be slowly tightened, taking several hours to sever the growth. If cut off quickly the bleeding may be fatal.

Destroying the tumor by cutting off small pieces is not advocated, as fatal hæmorrhage may result, and the frequent irritation may excite malignancy.

When not possible to reach the point of attachment, or, for any other reason the snare cannot be used, it is advisable to split the palate to gain access to the growth. Or, the operation of detaching the upper lip and nose from their attachment to the superior maxillary may be tried. (See article on Malignant Tumors of the Nose.) At the present day the external operations through the integument, for reaching the nasal space, are rarely if ever necessary.

ADENOIDS IN THE NASO-PHARYNX

Synonyms. Adenoid vegetations. Lymphoid hypertrophy in the naso-pharynx.

Definition. Adenoids may be designated as an hypertrophied condition of the lymphoid tissue in the naso-pharynx.

Etiology. In nearly all cases there will be found an underlying dyscrasia; the strumous diathesis is the most frequent.

It is claimed that the general depression following scarlet fever, diphtheria and sometimes measles, is a predisposing cause. This I believe to be true; but I also contend that the above-mentioned diseases are more severe, or malignant when attacking children with enlarged faucial and pharyngeal tonsils. It is claimed, and I believe with truth, that if children's noses and throats were kept in better condition there would be fewer severe throat complications in diphtheria, and fewer cases of otitis followed by otorrhœa in scarlet fever. From infancy the child should be taught to keep the nose clean by blowing; and the family physician should be permitted to care for existing lesions by proper internal or local measures, or both combined.

Symptoms. The symptoms are usually quite pronounced. The child catches cold at every change in the weather, especially in damp and cold weather. The patient always breathes through his mouth; this mouth-breathing is more noticeable during sleep, when the breathing is heavy and noisy. The child is restless during the night, and is apt to start, or cry out. These children frequently have so-called "night-terrors." The face is quite indicative of the condition. The mouth is open, the upper lip is thickened, the nose is pinched, the eyes are heavy. These characteristics give the child a stupid expression. Usually there is present some degree of deafness. In many cases there are recurring attacks of otitis, and not unfrequently otorrhœa. A hacking cough, which may be dry or moist, usually sets in during the early fall and continues until the beginning of summer. At times the frequent hacking becomes very annoying during sleep. Spasmodic croup is of frequent occurrence. Thoracic deformity, such as "pigeon-breast," many become pronounced. This is probably due to inability to properly inflate the lungs. The voice often has a peculiar deadness, or a thick muffled sound.

In many cases, also, the faucial tonsils are hypertrophied. Headache and chorea are among the neuroses that may be traced to adenoid growths.

Diagnosis. Rarely is the diagnosis attended with difficulty. In nearly all cases the symptoms point unmistakably to the trouble. Digital exploration will always verify the condition. If in a young child, place a wide tongue depressor edgewise between the teeth; in other children press the cheek between the teeth; then with the index finger of the other hand passed behind the free border of the soft palate, the enlargements are easily felt. (Fig. V, *c*.) To the touch they are soft, and the sensation elicited has been described as "feeling like a bunch of earth-worms." When the finger is withdrawn it is usually stained with bloody mucus. At times, in older patients, the growths are denser and more of a fibrous structure.

Prognosis. Some degree of improvement can be expected in nearly all cases.

After thorough removal of the tissue, the marked improvement that occurs in the child is often surprising.

It is my opinion, based upon a clinical experience, which is not altogether small, that few operations are so often followed by as satisfactory results as is that for the removal of adenoid growths. I desire, however, to emphasize the importance of removing all of the diseased tissue. It is true that atrophy of these growths often takes place in adult life; but, it is likewise true, that as these growths atrophy they give rise to cicatricial bands and cords on the pharyngeal vault, which frequently occlude the eustachian orifice and impair the integrity of the middle ear. This condition is one of the most prolific causes of tinnitus and deafness in the adult.

Treatment. While internal medication directed toward the constitutional bias is all important, surgical treatment is necessary in the vast majority of instances.

The growths are removed surgically in the following manner: after being anæsthetized the child is placed on its back, the head resting on the table; or, as some operators prefer, the head hanging over the end of the table. A mouth-gag is introduced, when the nasal space is examined with the finger to estimate the location and quantity of tissue to be removed. The soft palate is hooked forward with the finger, and the cutting forceps are introduced and as large a bite as possible secured. By cutting and twisting the tissue is removed. This is repeated until all the growth is brought away. The child is then quickly turned on its face, to permit the blood to escape from the nose and mouth. In the course of two or three minutes the anæsthetic is again given and remaining tags of tissue scraped with the curette or finger nail.

For removing the tissue on the lateral walls, the handle of the forceps, or curette, can be directed as necessary.

There are many varieties of forceps and curettes on the market; of the former I prefer Gradle's, or Brandage's modification of Gradle's. (Fig. X.) Its main

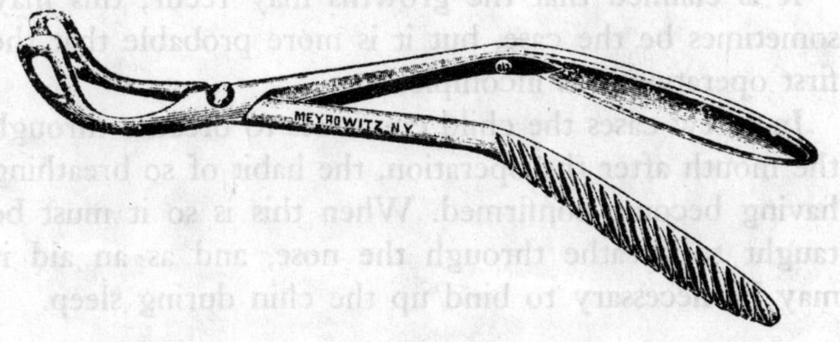

Fig. X

advantage is, the fenestra are curved so as to avoid catching the uvula. Of the many curettes, Gottestein's is the most useful. (Fig. XI.) Certain complications may fol-

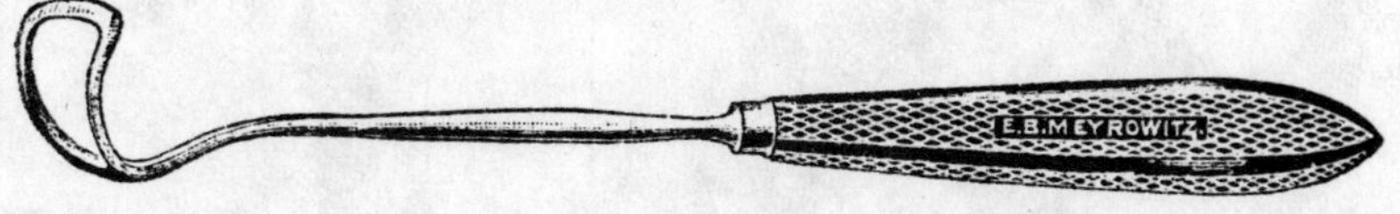

Fig. XI

low the operation; of these, acute otitis, caused by cutting the border of the eustachian orifice, or by blood entering the eustachian tubes, is the most common. The danger of blood entering the larynx is, I believe, overestimated; the child is more inclined to swallow the blood trickling down the throat than draw it into the windpipe.

If bleeding is severe, tampons of gauze pressed on the cut surface will usually be all that is necessary.

A few fatal cases have been reported, but the danger is no greater than in other operations where a general anæsthetic is used.

It is claimed that the growths may recur; this may sometimes be the case, but it is more probable that the first operation was incomplete.

In a few cases the child continues to breathe through the mouth after the operation, the habit of so breathing having become confirmed. When this is so it must be taught to breathe through the nose, and as an aid it may be necessary to bind up the chin during sleep.

Therapeutics

For a few weeks after the operation I usually prescribe one of the preparations of calcarea, iodine, or mercury, the choice of the remedy depending on the constitutional symptoms.

Chapter XIV

RETRO-PHARYNGEAL ABSCESS

Synonyms. Peri-pharyngeal abscess.

Definition. A retro-pharyngeal abscess is a collection of pus in the connective tissue between the pharynx and the vertebræ.

Etiology. It occurs principally in infants under one year of age. It is frequently the result of caries of the upper vertebræ in the scrofulous, tuberculous and syphilitic.

It may also be the result of acute pharyngitis. Likewise the septic infection of scarlet fever may produce it.

In infants an abscess of the tonsil may burrow and form collections of pus back of the pharynx. As the child usually lies on its back, and the connective tissue back of the tonsil is very loose, it can readily be seen that the tendency of the pus is to work toward the vertebræ.

When occurring in adults it is almost invariably caused by either syphilis or erysipelas. Occasionally it is due to a foreign body penetrating the pharyngeal wall during the act of swallowing.

During early life the glands at the second and third cervical vertebræ are quite large. This fact may account for the large abscesses that form in this locality as the result of suppuration.

Symptoms. When not due to traumatism the onset is slow. The child has a slight cough, and gradually there is difficult nasal respiration. There is pain on swallowing, and liquids regurgitate through the nose;

or, in passing downward, may enter the larynx.

With the formation of pus, there occur the usual chilly sensations, elevation of temperature and increased pulse. The neighboring glands enlarge, and tumefaction of the neck may be pronounced. The head is drawn to one side in an effort to relax the muscles; replacing the head causes severe pain.

Inspection of the parts will reveal congestion of the soft palate and tonsils. In the majority of cases the abscess is situated to one side of the median line, and frequently above the border of the soft palate. Or, it may be in the lower part of the pharynx. When situated in the latter place, the larynx becomes obstructed and severe dyspnœa with stertorous breathing ensues. This condition may be quickly followed by convulsions and death.

Diagnosis. The subjective symptoms may be mistaken for those due to croup or œdema of the larynx. Objectively the condition may simulate cerebral or digestive disorders.

In croup the cough has a metallic ring, and the voice is usually lost; there is no external swelling. From œdema of the larynx, the history of the case and a thorough inspection of the parts will prevent error in diagnosis. In œdema the difficulty in breathing comes suddenly; while in abscess the dyspnœa gradually increases.

Cerebral and digestive disorders, when ushered in by convulsions may, for a short time, simulate pharyngeal abscess. An examination of the pharynx will enable the physician to differentiate the two conditions.

There may be enlargement of the pharyngeal glands without suppuration.

When due to caries of the vertebræ the condition may exist for months, but usually terminates fatally. When not due to spondylitis recovery is the rule, the abscess rarely continuing longer than two weeks.

In many of the milder cases the abscess opens spontaneously. However, it is not always safe to trust to nature, as the pus may burrow down into the pharynx and death result from strangulation.

In many cases pneumonia is a complication, or it may closely follow the suppurative process.

Treatment. In children less than one year of age, when the abscess is in the median line, it should be opened internally. The knife is to be protected to within a half inch of the point. A longitudinal incision is to be made, and subsequently enlarged by introducing closed forceps into the abscess and withdrawing it with the blades separated.

Washing the cavity is rarely advisable, and hydrogen peroxide should never be injected into the sac.

Care must be exercised not to puncture the swelling before suppuration has occurred. When occurring on either side of the median line, in cases over one year of age, the external incision is to be preferred.

Two methods have been recommended. The first, by Chiene, is as follows: "To make an incision from the mastoid process down alongside the posterior border of the sterno-cleido-mastoid muscle, and then to go bluntly down with the finger and probe to the anterior aspect of the vertebral bodies. By dividing the deep fascia and retracting anteriorly the muscle with the complexity of vessels, the retro-pharyngeal space is quickly reached"

The other method is by Burckhart: "If one cuts down at a level with the larynx, on the inner side of the sterno-cleido-mastoid muscle, through skin and platysma, the vessels of the thyroid gland are first encountered (a larger or smaller subcutaneous vein, which may communicate with the thyroid vessels, is to be caught between two artery forceps, cut and ligated). Between them on the outer, and the larynx on the inner side, the inner border of the common carotid is quckly exposed by blunt dissection. As no branches are here given off from the main trunk one may safely make, in the depth, an incision with the knife just at the side of the larynx, or rather the lower end of the pharynx, into the thickened tissue, which is generally found here in these cases on account of the neighboring purulent inflammation. If this incision is then enlarged, by opening the branches of a slender dressing-forceps or similar instrument, the retro-pharyngeal space is fully and easily accessible."

Therapeutics

Internally the remedies usually indicated in pus formation are to be given.

Chapter XV

TONSILLITIS

Synonyms. Catarrhal tonsillitis. Angina faucium. Lacunar or follicular tonsillitis. Amygdalitis.

Definition. Tonsillitis signifies an acute inflammation of the mucous membrane covering the tonsils; or the inflammation may involve the whole gland; or, it may implicate the gland and the surrounding tissue.

Clinically the disease may be divided into three varieties:

Lacunar or follicular tonsillitis, characterized by superficial inflammation of the mucous membrane covering the tonsil, and with white or yellowish exudation issuing from the tonsil crypts; both tonsils may be affected, but generally one more severely than the other.

Parenchymatous tonsillitis, when the whole gland, usually on one side, is inflamed, which may be followed by suppuration.

Peritonsillitis or Quinsy, when the gland and surrounding connective tissue is involved, and usually resulting in suppuration; this variety is commonly unilateral.

Etiology. During the fall and spring months inflammation of the tonsils is of common occurrence. It oftener attacks children or young people with enlarged faucial and pharyngeal tonsils. The first attack usually occurs between the twelfth and the fifteen year of age, although the disease is frequently seen in infants and young children.

There is a marked hereditary tendency. One attack

predisposes to another; these may occur yearly, or at varying intervals until the fortieth year of age, yet the disease is not infrequent in advanced life.

The exciting cause is usually exposure to cold, damp or changeable weather, especially if the state of health is below par and there exists derangement of the digestive organs.

During certain seasons lacunar tonsillitis appears to be epidemic and is frequently eminently infectious; it is not unusual to find succeeding cases in the same family suffering with this form of tonsillitis, a few days after the advent of the first.

Unsanitary dwellings and exposure to septic conditions, either in the house or in the open air, are undoubtedly exciting causes. Diphtheria, scarlet fever and measles are usually ushered in with catarrhal inflammation of the tonsils; likewise syphilitic manifestations in the pharynx show some degree of tonsillar inflammation.

When the predisposition is present, amenorrhœa is occasionally followed by tonsillitis.

Symptoms. The disease is usually ushered in with chilliness, oppressive headache, dryness and stinging, darting pain in the throat, aching in the back and limbs. In the lacunar form, during the first twenty-four to forty-eight hours, a light yellowish exudation makes its appearance at the openings of the tonsillar crypts; in some cases the exudation is so abundant that, by coalition, it covers a large surface of the exposed gland. In nearly all cases the exudation can easily be rubbed off, yet occasionally it is strongly adherent, and when rubbed, or pulled off, it leaves a raw surface.

When the inflammation implicates the gland structure and the surrounding tissue, the headache, pains in the back and limbs, and stinging pain in the throat become intensified. The tongue is thickly covered with a white or yellowish, moist coating, the breath is exceedingly fetid, there is a profuse flow of thick saliva; on account of the intense pain in swallowing, the patient inclines his head forward to permit the saliva to dribble out.

The faucial pillars are inflamed and the uvula may be decidedly œdematous, presenting a bluish water-soaked condition. Frequently the fauces are so blocked up by the inflammation, and infiltration of the tissues, that there is barely space to permit the air to pass into the larynx.

There is frequently complete inability to swallow food, and when an attempt is made to drink the liquid may be ejected through the nostrils. The sense of taste is blunted, probably because of the foul covering on the tongue. Pain in the ear, due to extension of the inflammation along the eustachian tube is frequently present. Speech is painful and may be almost unintelligible. The glands under the angle of the lower jaw are enlarged, there is always high fever present and it is not uncommon for the temperature to reach 105° F.

Diagnosis. Clinically the disease to which tonsillitis bears the closest resemblance is diphtheria. It is advisable to make it a rule that when children complain of sore throat, with inflammation and deposit on the tonsil, they should be isolated and considered as suspected diphtheritic cases until a clear diagnosis can be made.

In tonsillitis the attack is more acute than in diphtheria; during the first thirty-six hours the thermometer may reach 104° F.; in diphtheria during the same period it will seldom register above 101 degrees, and may be sub-normal, but later in the attack, when decided sepsis is present, the fever is quite high. Tonsillitis is rarely ushered in by vomiting and nose-bleed; diphtheria frequently is.

In tonsillitis the deposit is not likely to extend beyond one or both tonsils; in diphtheria the tendency is for the membrane to spread over the soft palate, uvula, posterior nares and the nostrils. In tonsillitis the exudation first appears in isolated spots; these may join and cover a large surface of the tonsil, but the exudation does not present the firm appearance of diphtheria membrane.

The time-honored distinction usually quoted, that when the exudation due to tonsillitis is rubbed off it does not leave a bleeding surface, but that when the membrane due to diphtheria is pulled off, the contrary is the case, does not in my experience hold true. I believe that time will demonstrate this test to be unreliable.

In tonsillitis it is frequently impossible for the patient to open his mouth, so as to present a view of the fauces; in the more serious disease this is rarely so. Tonsillitic patients may have albumen in the urine; those suffering with diphtheria invariably have.

Both diseases have enlarged glands under the angle of the jaw. In diphtheria the odor is *sui generis*.

It must be remembered that many cases of lacunar tonsillitis septic in origin are diphtheritic in character. The ability to determine whether the disease is tonsillitis or a mild form of diphtheria is not as sinple as it is usually considered to be.

Prognosis. In the lacunar form the acute inflammation terminates in five or six days. When the deeper structures are involved with formation of abscess, the disease usually continues seven to twelve days, and may be prolonged twenty-one days. Cases proving fatal have been reported where the abscess burrowed into the larynx.

It is also claimed that death has resulted from the inflamed tonsils completely blocking up the air passages. Were I to meet with this complication, I should deem amputation of the inflamed tonsils a justifiable procedure. Rheumatism with cardiac implication occasionally follows the lacunar form.

Treatment. In the lacunar variety, when possible, the exudation should be removed from the surface of the tonsil and the crypts emptied of their contents. For this purpose there is nothing better than a spray of peroxide of hydrogen applied by means of an air condenser of twenty to twenty-five pounds pressure. With the curved tip of the atomizer tube the space between the tonsil and the lateral pillars, and the crypts in the tonsils, are freed of all accumulations. The quantity of fetid *detritus* that will be expelled is surprising. In the absence of an air condenser, a hand atomizer with a long, hard-rubber tube can be used. A small curette, or if that is not covenient, a metal applicator with one end properly curved, will answer for cleaning the crypts, but it is not as satisfactory as a spray.

During the past few years I have used in these cases, with decided benefit, the galvano-cautery electrode.

The platinum point, heated to a dull-red color, is carried (for about one-half inch) into five to eight crypts in each tonsil. In my experience with the cauterization the majority of cases treated within the first thirty-six hours will be quickly aborted.

Of course, in treating young children, it is frequently impossible to use local applications; reliance must then be placed on the internal remedy.

When the inflammation progresses to the formation of an abscess, the application of a hot flax-seed poultice every one to two hours, on the neck, over the enlarged gland, or bag of hot, moist hops, may be used; this will aid pus formation and also serve to relax the infiltrated tissues.

If the pain caused by gargling is not too severe, a solution for this purpose, of either carbolic acid or of capsicum, ten drops to four ounces of hot water, is soothing. I believe that steam inhalations, so frequently recommended, cause relaxation of the mucous membrane, and frequently œdema; after their use it is not infrequent to find either bronchial or lung inflammation. The temporary relief afforded by sucking ice is followed by increased dryness of the mucous membrane; the same result follows the application of cocaine.

For the intense thirst which is usually present, sips of very hot water are grateful. As acids antidote aconite and kali permanganate, acidulated drinks must not be used when these remedies are prescribed. Constipation being an invariable accompaniment, a thorough rectal flushing is advisable.

It is an axiom in surgery, that an abscess should be opened to permit the evacuation of pus. I believe a tonsillar abscess is not an exception to the rule. By timely and proper opening the patient usually is saved days of suffering. A small incision is liable to close before the abscess is thoroughly free from pus, thus necessitating subsequent openings. On the other hand, by using a sharp-pointed, curved bistoury (keeping the cutting edge toward the median line) and carrying the blade deeply into the tonsil, one or two free incisions permit the free evacuation of pus. The points to remember are, insert the blade well back of the anterior pillar, being careful not to cut its free border, and cut toward the median line of the mouth.

Therapeutics

Guaiacum. When given early in the lx dilution, twenty drops in a half glass of water, one teaspoonful every half hour for three hours, then every one or two hours, it will frequently cut short or modify an attack. "Violent burning and pricking in the throat, with thirst and dryness of the mouth; constant violent stitches in the throat. Especially adapted to complaints founded on a rheumatic or rheumatico-syphilitic diathesis."

Kali permanganate. Has been claimed to prevent suppuration, two grains to one ounce of boiled water. When using this drug absolutely no form of acids nor sweets are allowed, as they antidote its medicinal action. This remedy gives excellent results when used as a mouth wash, also as a spray on the tonsils.

Belladonna. Fauces and tonsils deep red; mucous membrane very dry; constant desire to swallow, feels as if he would choke if he did not; the act of swallowing is very painful; liquids may be ejected through the nose.

Throbbing headache, and even delirium.

Capsicum. Constriction of the throat; smarting, burning blisters. The free border of the soft palate painful when swallowing.

Phytolacca. Frequently indicated during epidemics. Great aching, feeling as if pounded all over. Fauces dry, congested, and of a dark, or of a bluish-red color; metallic taste in the mouth. When swallowing shooting pains through both ears. Feels as if a hot ball, or a lump were in the throat. Swelling of the sublingual glands. Patient subject to rheumatism, or the pains of a rheumatic character. When the effort is not too severe, a gargle of the tincture, twenty drops to four ounces of water, is sufficient.

Mercurius bin. Painful swelling of the submaxillary glands. Fetid saliva, which causes constant swallowing; large, flabby tongue; elongation of uvula. Throbbing in tonsil, sticking pain in fauces when swallowing. When suppuration begins, secretion from the mouth is slimy, stringy, with great fetor. Pain worse on empty swallowing.

Mercurius cor. It is claimed that this remedy in the lx trituration, applied locally to the tonsil, will arrest suppuration.

Lachesis. Neck sensitive to contact, or to pressure. Uvula elongated, fauces purplish; small, circumscribed spots of dryness in the throat; constant desire to swallow, or a sensation of a lump in the throat, which needs to be swallowed. Solid food swallowed easier than liquids, which are apt to escape through the nose. Invariably worse after sleeping.

Ammonium carb. Great dryness in mouth and throat;

pain in mouth, as if raw. Feels as if mouth were swollen. Free flow of saliva. Tendency to ulceration. Feels as if something had lodged in the throat when swallowing.

Apis. Tonsils swollen bright red; stinging, burning pains. Soft palate and uvula œdematous, looks water-soaked. Blisters on back part of throat. Tenacious, dirty, grayish mucus.

Baptisia. Tongue heavily coated; salivation; putrid, offensive breath. Uvula elongated; fauces dark red. Can swallow liquids easier than solids. Jaws may be firmly closed.

Hepar sulph. cal. Glandular swelling of neck. Lancinating pain, as if caused by splinters in the throat, especially when swallowing. Difficult deglutition; pressure in throat with danger of suffocation. Throbbing in tonsils, fetid breath, metallic taste. Great chilliness, sensitive to open air; sweats from slight motion.

When suppuration is inevitable, this remedy, given in the 2x trituration, will assist pus formation, but as soon as pus begins to discharge, if this remedy be continued, it should be given in the higher potencies.

HYPERTROPHY OF THE TONSILS

Etiology. Chronic enlargement of the tonsils is generally seen in children, although the condition is frequent in adults.

A scrofulous constitution predisposes to glandular enlargement. The hypertrophied condition frequently results from repeated attacks of tonsillitis, and acute pharyngitis.

It is also a frequent result of diphtheria and scarlet fever. The hard, fibrous tonsil is usually produced by repeated attacks of acute tonsillar inflammation.

Symptoms. The voice is unusually thick and nasal. Respiration is often laborious, especially at night. Snoring and starting during sleep are common. Head-colds and sore throat are of frequent occurrence. The hearing is often impaired, especially when adenoid tissue is also present. A dry, hacking cough is frequent, due to contact of the enlarged tonsils with the surrounding tissue. Or, it may be due to increased secretion.

Children with enlarged tonsils usually drink after each mouthful of food, as it is often difficult for the child to swallow without the aid of liquid.

When occurring in infants, nursing is quite difficult.

In many cases secretion of cheesy character presents at the mouth of the crypts. The exudation is usually extremely fetid. When the enlargement is the result of acute tonsillitis the gland is generally attached to the lateral pillars. When hypertrophy of the tonsils is present before the age of puberty, acute tonsillitis is apt to occur during that period.

Prognosis. Tonsillar hypertrophy in itself is not dangerous to life. However, the existing complications may excite serious disorders of the respiratory tract. Furthermore, the enlarged tonsil with its roughened surface offers a seat of lodgment for particles of food and foreign bodies, which may set up a septic condition.

Treatment. The treatment is both medical and surgical. In many cases the best results are obtained by employing both. When the enlarged tonsils fail to yield to internal medication, and it is evident that they interfere with the health of the patient, I believe it is then the duty of the physician to excise them. It is claimed that the tonsils are physiological organs and should not be removed. This argument is hardly a valid one when they fail in performing their functions and are a menace to health; no stronger proof of the utility of the question, when indicated, can be produced than that it is invariably followed by improved health. Facts adduced outweigh all theories.

For removing the tonsils in children the Mackenzie (Fig. XII), or the Mathieu tonsillotome without the

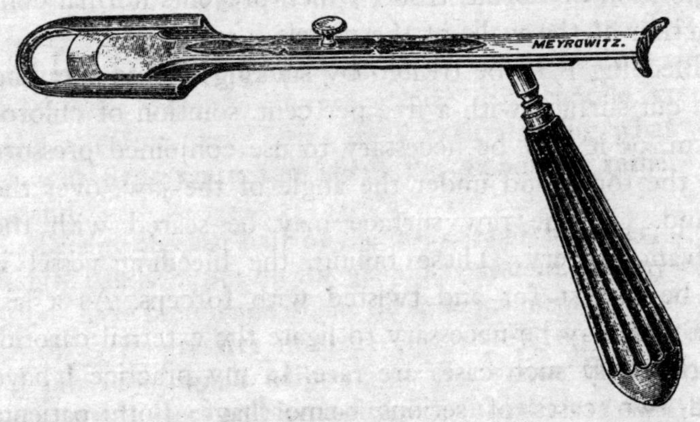

Fig. XII

barbs on the spear-points are to be preferred. Directed by a strong light the fenestra of the instrument is carried around the tonsil back to the border of the pillars. Pressure is then made on the shaft of the blade. The excised piece comes off, adhering to the instrument. Where the tonsil and pillars are attached they must be first separated by a curved probe, or by the finger. Often the tonsil is enlarged vertically; when such is the case it may be necessary to take it off in two pieces.

The operation is nearly painless, but in children a general anæsthetic may be required to control the patient.

I believe cocaine injected into the gland tends to cause secondary hæmorrhage.

Bleeding after tonsillotomy usually ceases in a few minutes, but cases occur where it becomes severe.

The causes are (1) hæmophillia; (2) abnormality in the distribution of the blood vessels; and (3) unnatural deposition of fibrous tissue, which prevents normal contraction of the walls of the vessels.

Bleeding is to be treated by sucking ice, or spraying the cut surface with a five per cent. solution of chloroform, or it may be necessary to use conjoined pressure on the tonsil and under the angle of the jaw, over the gland. Or, the raw surface may be seared with the galvano-cautery. These failing, the bleeding vessel is to be sought for and twisted with forceps. As a last resort it may be necessary to ligate the external carotid. Fortunately such cases are rare. In my practice I have had two cases of serious hæmorrhage. Both patients were "bleeders." In the first, various styptics were employed without benefit, but the bleeding ceased immediately on using a chloroform spray; in the second case, a little girl eight years of age, both tonsils were amputated and mass of adenoid tissue removed at one operation. After some hours spent in vain effort to stay the oozing, I used the same spray with equally good result. One patient was confined to his room four, and the other six weeks. In neither instance did I enquire before operating, as I should have done, whether or not the bleeding tendency was present. When aware of the existence of the hæmorrhagic diathesis I never operate.

When tonsillar hypertrophy occurs in adults, or in children, when the tonsillotome cannot be used, the enlarged gland may be cut off with the cold-wire snare, or the galvano-cautery snare. Or, the cautery point can be used, the platinum being pressed into the crypt for one-half inch. The point is then heated to a cherry-red and slowly withdrawn. The current is not turned on until the electrode is inserted into the crypt. Nor should it be turned off until the point has been withdrawn from the tonsil.

Each tonsil is punctured three or four times at each sitting. The treatment should be given about once a week. Six to ten treatments will usually reduce the largest tonsil.

The operator must guard against touching the lateral pillars or the tongue with the hot electrode.

Puncturing the tonsil with nitrate of silver has been recommended. Benefit may sometimes result from swabbing the tonsil with iodine once a day.

The various escharotic pastes that produce sloughing should never be applied to the tonsils.

Provided the child is under a general anæsthetic, adenoid vegetations, when present, can be removed at the same time; but the tonsils should first be excised, as their removal will permit of greater space for the post-nasal operation.

During the prevalence of an epidemic it is not wise to operate.

For three or four days after amputating the tonsils, the diet should be restricted to bland, liquid, or semi-solid food. Nothing of a dry or coarse character is to be eaten, as such articles of food are apt to irritate the cut surface, thus causing secondary hæmorrhage.

The use of the voice and active exercise are to be prohibited for a few days.

Therapeutics

Baryta mur. Enlarged tonsils, smooth and deeply cleft by sulci.

Calcarea carb. Dilated veins on soft palate. The constitutional symptoms are the main indications, late dentition, light hair, protuberant abdomen, etc.

Calcarea phos. Pale, flabby hypertrophy of tonsils. General malnutrition; emaciated. Scrofulous diathesis.

Mercurius bin. Tongue and gums swollen; profuse discharge of saliva. Frequent acute inflammation of tonsils. Breath fetid.

Phytolacca. Tonsils bluish-red, feels as if a lump lodged in throat.

Consult *Ignatia*, *Lycopodium*, *Psorinum* and *Sulphur*.

TONSILLAR CALCULI

Concretions in the tonsils are a result of closure of the openings of the crypts. When the mass has been retained for some time it becomes hard and of a calcareous formation. They do not always produce disturbance, yet at times they may aid in causing tonsillitis.

The *treatment* consists in seizing the concretion with forceps and pulling it out. When bands of tissue prevent it being dragged out, they are to be cut with scissors or knife. A calculus may be so deeply imbedded in the gland as to interfere with the knife during tonsillotomy.

HYPERTROPHY OF THE LINGUAL TONSIL

Etiology. Hypertrophy of the glands on the base of the tongue is commonly found just prior to the age of puberty. Or, they may enlarge during adult life. Usually the neurotic temperament is well marked.

Symptoms. The subjective symptoms are of a foreign body in the throat, which causes the patient to cough in an effort to remove the obstruction. Or, the sensation in the throat may be of a tickling character.

Deglutition at times may be difficult, owing to the sense of obstruction.

Examination with the laryngoscope will reveal the glands enlarged, and frequently in contact with the epiglottis.

Prognosis. The prognosis is invariably good.

Treatment. The treatment should be directed toward relieving any predisposing constitutional conditions present.

Daily swabbing the glands with iodine crystals, two grains, to glycerine, one ounce, will often aid in reducing them.

If this fail, the glands should be pierced with the galvano-cautery point, as directed under "Follicular Pharyngitis."

LINGUAL VARIX

Symptoms. Occasionally there is seen a varicose condition on the base of the tongue. They may give rise to the various symptoms produced by hypertrophy of the lingual glands. In addition, they not infrequently rupture, the discharged blood being mistaken for plumonary bleeding. But the use of the laryngoscope will show the point of rupture. Several years ago Dr. Passmore Berens called my attention to the co-existence of anal hæmorrhoids with lingual varix, a condition that I have since repeatedly verified.

Treatment. The treatment consists in the local application of hamamelis. Or, when this fails, the enlarged veins are to be punctured with the galvano-cautery point.

Therapeutics

Consult *Hamamelis*, *Collinsonia* and *Nux vomica.*

DISEASES OF THE UVULA

Elongation or relaxed uvula, with relaxation of the soft palate, is common as the result of chronic pharyngitis. The uvula resting on the back of the tongue, causes a frequent desire to clear the throat; in the recumbent position the irritation is on the posterior wall of the pharynx. As a result of the constant efforts to clear the throat, sleep is disturbed, and frequently the general health suffers.

The *treatment* consists in applying to one ounce of water an astringent solution of alum, twenty grains; sulphate of zinc, ten grains; or tannin, fifteen grains. When local applications fail, amputation of the lower end is necessary. This may be accomplished by a uvulatome. Or, in the absence of a special instrument, the tip of the uvula is grasped by forceps, gently pulled forward and cut off with a pair of scissors, curved on the flat, with the convexity below.

To properly amputate the uvula is sometimes a difficult matter, as the tendency is for the patient to draw the uvula up as soon as it is caught with forceps. Unless care is exercised it may be severed too close to its attachment to the palate. For from one to three days afterward there is sharp pain on swallowing. This can usually be relieved by gargling hot milk or water.

Papillomata and angeiomata on the end of the uvula are occcasionally met with. The treatment consists in amputating the uvula above the seat of the growths.

Bi-fid, split and fish-tail uvulæ do not require treatment unless they interfere with vocalization.

Berens, in three thousand throats examined, found eighty-four cases where the uvula presented some anomaly. They are classified as follows:

Completely separate	2
Worm-like shreds	8
Supernumerary	4
Deeply cleft	14
Attached to other parts	2
Absence	2
Fish-tail shaped	39
Pendulum	2
Hypertrophied	11

Chapter XVI

ACUTE CATARRHAL LARYNGITIS

Synonyms. Laryngeal hyperæmia.

Etiology. Acute laryngitis is usually limited to an inflammatory condition of the mucous membrane. A severer form is produced by acute infectious diseases or typhoid fever. Or, it may be caused by direct violence. In the idiopathic form the various conditions embraced under "taking cold" are the most prominent causes, especially sudden exposure to cold when overheated. In this climate the sudden changes occurring during the fall and spring months are productive of acute laryngitis. The condition may also be produced by inhaling irritating vapors, dust, etc., through the mouth. One attack predisposes to another. Frequent recurring attacks of acute laryngitis are often a forerunner of laryngeal tuberculosis. In some persons acute rhinitis always terminates in catarrhal laryngitis.

Symptoms. The inflammation may come on gradually, or, in severe attacks, the first symptom being a chill quickly followed by elevated temperature. Burning and itching in the larynx are usually present. The throat is painful to pressure, with a feeling of tightness or constriction. The voice is hoarse, soon becoming aphonic. Cough is dry with sense of tearing in the throat. As exudation occurs, expectoration may be quite profuse. In children the cough is of a barking, croupy character; respiration may become painful and rapid.

Prognosis. This condition lasts ordinarily from two

days to two weeks. A neglected case is apt to run into the chronic form.

Laryngeal œdema is a possible complication.

En passant, a word in relation to traditional medicine.

One of the physicians in attendance records that, "George Washington died of acute laryngitis, after one day's illness. His treatment consisted in drawing from his veins one quart of blood; in two hours a pint of blood was again drawn. In five hours his condition was no better and he was again bled. This time the blood ran slowly, appeared very thick, and did not produce any symptoms of fainting. In addition, fly-blisters were applied to his throat and to his legs. Calomel and tartar emetic were given internally."

In children the prognosis must be guarded, as laryngeal œdema, and in some cases pneumonia, may be a complication.

In alcoholism the disease is much more fatal than in persons not addicted to liquors. In chronic drunkards the mortality is fully ninety per cent.

Diagnosis. The acute laryngitis of syphilis is to be distinguished by the history of the case and the syphilitic symptoms.

Treatment. In all cases, but especially in severe attacks, the patient should be kept in bed. Plenty of fresh air is necessary, but draughts must be avoided.

Copious rectal enemata are often beneficial.

Steam inhalations are recommended as aids in lessening the hoarseness and relieving cough. Inhalations are to continue for from five to fifteen minutes and repeated every one to three hours. The water should be about 140 degrees Fahrenheit. During the early stage, for relieving the pain, tincture of benzoin, ten drops, to one ounce water; or, chloroform, five drops, added to the benzoin is soothing. Or, inhalation of equal parts of vinegar and water is useful.

Therapeutics

Aconite. First stage; short, dry cough. Larynx sensitive to touch and to inspired air. Great anxiety and restlessness, with fever. Also after straining the voice.

Ammonium carb. "Hoarseness, cannot speak a loud word; aggravation from speaking; great dryness. Larynx as if drawn shut from both sides of throat."

Belladonna. Sudden œdematous swelling of larynx. Constriction and great dryness of larynx. Aphonia; dry cough; vocal cords bright red. Face flushed, throbbing headache; over-excitability.

Ferrum phos. First stage. Similar to *Aconite*, but without the anxiety and restlessness.

Guaiacum. Burning sensation in larynx, with palpitation of heart.

Iodium. Hoarseness, tightness and soreness about larynx. Cough dry, croupy character.

Phosphorus. Great rawness in the larynx, with dry, hacking cough. Aphonia, larynx sensitive to pressure. Blood-streaked expectoration. Talking aggravates all the symptoms.

Consult *Causticum*, *Rumex* and *Sanguinaria*.

CHRONIC LARYNGITIS

Synonyms. Chronic laryngeal catarrh.

Etiology. Chronic inflammation of the larynx may result from repeated attacks of acute laryngitis. Or, it may be caused by the various forms of chronic inflammation implicating the nose and pharynx. Digestive derangements and disorders of the genitalia are frequent causes. Likewise the etiological factors productive of chronic pharyngitis apply equally well to chronic laryngitis.

As a rule, chronic laryngitis is insidious in its development.

Symptoms. The pronounced objective symptom is a change in the timbre of the voice. This may be constant, or as is more often the case, there is a huskiness in cold and changeable weather with amelioration in summer. Or, there may be complete aphonia. In singers the range of voice is materially restricted.

A sense of dryness, rawness, and burning in the throat is frequently present. Cough is not always complained of, but there is a frequent desire to clear the throat.

Secretion is rarely free, but at times small pellets of mucus are suddenly expelled from the mouth when coughing.

On inspection with the laryngoscope portions of the membrane appear redder than normal; or, spots of erosion are seen, especially in the arytenoid space. Small strings of mucus are found on the bands and vocal cords; these frequently extend across the orifice of the glottis.

In singers and professional voice-users small nodes are frequently present on the inner margins of the vocal cords.

The cords may be nearly normal in color, or present congested spots, or have the appearance of raw beef.

Prognosis. Recovery is always slow. Faithfulness in treatment should be insisted upon.

When the tissues have become infiltrated restoration of the voice is not to be expected.

Ulcers on the cords and swelling of the cartilages of Santorini and Wrisberg are strongly suspicious of tuberculosis.

Treatment. The treatment, to be beneficial, implies the discovery and removal of all predisposing and exciting causes.

A change of climate is often decidedly beneficial. For inland patients a prolonged residence at the seashore is frequently followed by great relief.

Nasal and pharyngeal disorders should be relieved. Likewise improper vocalization should be corrected. Due attention should be given to all hygienic measures, as diet, exercise and wearing proper clothing. Woollen undergarments should be worn during all seasons of the year.

Local treatment is of prime importance and consists, first, in cleansing the membrane; and, second, applying remedial agents. The secretions are best removed by alkaline spray, borax being one of the most useful, four grains to water one ounce; or, if fetor be present, permanganate of potash, one to three grains, to water one ounce. After the membrane is cleansed one of the following stimulating applications to the dried mucous membrane may be used; chloride of potash, five grains, or carbolic acid, two grains, to water one ounce.

Where the secretion is profuse a spray of hydrogen peroxide, one part to water three parts, is useful. Inhalations of the vapor of nascent chloride of ammonia is also useful. Spots of ulceration may be touched with a cotton-wrapped applicator dipped in one of the following solutions: chloride of zinc, five to ten grains, to water one ounce; or perchloride of iron, two to five grains, to water one ounce.

Nodes on the cords are to be removed by the curette, or by applying the preceding zinc, or iron solutions.

Therapeutics

Ammonium mur. "Hoarseness, with burning in larynx, afternoon. Frequent hawking, with expectoration of small lumps of mucus and sensation of rawness in throat."

Antimonium crud. "Loss of voice from getting overheated."

Argentum met. Hoarseness, especially of professional speakers and singers. "Expectoration of lumps of clear mucus, like boiled starch."

Arsenicum alb. Laryngeal mucous membrane dirty-red or anæmic. Burning in larynx; voice husky and trembles; fatigue from speaking.

Calcarea carb. Dry, tickling cough, aggravated by speaking. Mucous membrane of larynx thickened. Painless hoarseness; voice weak. Discharge of jelly-like, or tough mucus, may taste sweetish.

Causticum. Mucous membrane dry, glazed. Inability to speak a loud word because cords do not come together. Loss of voice from overexertion. When attempting to produce a high note voice ends in a squeak.

Gelsemium. Hoarseness, with aphonia. Cough excited when any part of the body gets cold, Muco-purulent expectoration; aggravated by overuse of the voice.

Kali bich. Rough, hoarse voice. Tickling in larynx, extending to mouth and ears. Mucous membrane dark red. Ulceration and necrosis of cartilages. Varicose veins in throat. Expectoration stringy, tough, like white of egg.

Kali nit. Tightness in larynx. Frequent, dry, short, hacking cough, with roughness in throat.

Lachesis. Larynx sensitive to touch. Hoarseness; sensation of something in larynx that cannot be hawked up, although mucus is expectorated. Feeling of something swollen in pit of the throat. Aggravation after sleep.

Mercurius cor. "Cutting in throat as from a knife."

Phosphorus. "Hoarseness and loss of voice, worse in evening; cannot talk on account of pain in larynx." Larynx sensitive and dry, feeling as if lined with fur. Aphonia from loud talking. Cough worse coming from a warm room into cold air.

(I believe this remedy is oftener prescribed than it is indicated.)

Rhus tox. Hoarseness from overstraining the voice. Cold sensation in larynx when breathing.

Rumex. Constant desire to hawk tenacious mucus in larynx. Raw sensation in throat. Hacking, spasmodic cough, coming from low down in the larynx. Aggravated by inhaling cold air and at night.

Sanguinaria. Aphonia; dryness; soreness in throat. Expectoration of thick mucus. Incipient pulmonary consumption.

Senega. Short, hacking cough in the open air. Great dryness in the throat, with oppression in the chest.

Stannum. Hoarseness and roughness in larynx. Voice

hoarse, deep; aphonia; beginning of laryngeal tuberculosis.

Thuja. Sensation as of a skin in the larynx.

ŒDEMA OF THE LARYNX

Synonyms. Œdema of the glottis. Phlegmonous laryngitis.

Etiology. Œdema of the larynx may result from swallowing corrosive liquids, from inhaling acrid vapors, or may be caused by traumatism.

It may result from diphtheria or the exanthemata, and it is a frequent complication of syphilis, tuberculosis and cancer of the larynx. Laryngeal œdema may be induced by inflammation of adjacent structures. It is occasionally met with in pyæmia and Bright's disease. Likewise it may be a part of a general dropsical condition.

Symptoms. Pain and increasing dyspnœa are the most prominent. The cough is hoarse and croupous, and swallowing is painful.

As the œdema progresses expiration becomes difficult and all the symptoms become intensified. The patient struggles for breath, a cold perspiration breaks out on the face and the skin becomes purplish. Unless relieved, coma and asphyxia speedily ensue.

The laryngoscope will reveal the infiltrated tissues, presenting a watery and translucent appearance. This is decidedly marked in the epiglottis, which looks like a large puffy tumor; the ary-epiglottic folds appear puffy and somewhat oval in shape.

In the absence of a mirror digital exploration will serve to diagnose the condition. This is accomplished by pulling the tongue well forward and introducing the index finger of the other hand into the mouth, when the boggy condition is easily recognized.

Prognosis. When the condition is acute and the effusion is a secondary result, the prognosis must be guarded.

But if œdema is limited to a portion of the larynx, and is caused by inflammation of the pharynx, the prognosis is more hopeful.

As relapses are frequent, great care must be exercised for several weeks after apparent recovery.

In chronic cases the prognosis necessarily depends on the cause.

Treatment. The temperature of the room should be kept at 70 to 72° F.

Relief may follow inhalations of steam containing tincture benzoin, ten to fifteen drops, and water one ounce. If the dyspnœa increases, scarification of the œdematous tissue is demanded. This may be accomplished by using a sharp-pointed curved bistoury wrapped with cotton or plaster to within one-half inch of the point. Several punctures will liberate the effused liquid. This will often be followed by decided amelioration.

If these methods fail to give relief, intubation, or low tracheotomy must be performed.

Pilocarpine, one-sixth grain hypodermically, has been followed by favorable results.

Therapeutics

Apis. Sudden attacks resulting from erysipelas, or fever; or caused by burns.

Arsenicum. A general anasarca the result of cardiac or kidney disease.

Kali iod. Syphilitic œdema.

Consult *Bromine, Iodine* and *Sanguinaria.*

Chapter XVII

SYPHILITIC PHARYNGITIS AND LARYNGITIS

The secondary and tertiary lesions only of syphilis will be considered.

Symptoms. The secondary manifestations of syphilis in the throat are not always characteristic of the disease. There is commonly a sense of dryness in the throat, and with this there may be a slight rise in temperature. In the beginning of this stage there is usually a uniform redness of the throat, which soon disappears from a large part of the surface but leaves well-defined patches of redness on corresponding parts of both sides, generally upon the pillars, and which extends up to the uvula; in some cases the redness may be pronounced on the soft palate. Mucous patches in the mouth are characteristic. The voice is impaired and there is some degree of hoarseness. Cough and pain are frequently absent. However, in some cases there is dyspnœa and pain in the act of swallowing. During this stage there are usually papillary eruptions upon the skin, but in some instances the only evidences of secondary syphilis are tc be seen in the larynx.

The tertiary form of the disease often causes ulceration without the patient being aware of the destruction of tissue. The *gummata* rarely causes inconvenience, unless interfering with the act of swallowing. They appear as small nodules beneath the mucous membrane, which gradually enlarge; they then soften and present a yellow spot at their center. This gives way and is followed by the characteristic clear-cut, deep, indurated syphilitic ulcer. Their bases are usually covered with a foul, purulent secretion, which when wiped off shows the floors of the ulcers to be covered with small granulations. A deep ulcer on the palate quickly tends to perforation. Tertiary syphilis in the larynx is accompanied by impairment of voice. In severe cases this is followed by difficult breathing, which is usually worse at night.

The epiglottis becomes infiltrated, its borders present a cockscomb, or a punched-out appearance, and it may be depressed in various ways. Occasionally it is perforated. Or, it may be reduced to a mere stump. Not infrequently the ulceration extends along the ary-epiglottic folds.

Patches of erythema on the vocal cords are quite characteristic of syphilis. If the ulceration continues chondritis and perichondritis ensue. Syphilitic ulcers tend to heal from the periphery.

Diagnosis. Syphilitic ulcers are preceded by *gummata*, and develop rapidly. The ulcer is surrounded by an inflammatory areola. Occasionally cicatricial contractions may be seen. The breath has a peculiarly fetid odor, and evidences of syphilitic rhinitis are frequently present. The history of the case and other symptoms of syphilis may be present. Syphilitic ulceration tends to work downward. Cervical enlargement is frequent. The pain is usually of a dull character.

When the diagnosis is in doubt, anti-syphilitic treatment should always be tried.

In tuberculosis the ulcers are sluggish, the surrounding mucous membrane is paler. The respiration is always, more or less, embarrassed. The temperature is increased and the pulse quickened. Tuberculous ulceration usually works upward. (See Laryngeal Tuberculosis.)

Cancer is a disease which occurs usually after the fortieth year. Lancinating pain, radiating to the ear, is common. Infiltration and ulceration are usually confined to one locality. As the tissue breaks down hæmorrhages are common. A microscopical examination may aid in the diagnosis.

Prognosis. In secondary syphilis the prognosis is good, although the singing voice may be permanently impaired. In the tertiary stage the result is usually satisfactory, unless cicatricial contraction causing deformity and interfering with the functions of the larynx result. Destruction of the cartilages is always a serious matter. Intubation, or tracheotomy, may be demanded to save life.

Treatment. (See Syphilitic Rhinitis.)

Chapter XVIII

LARYNGEAL TUBERCULOSIS

Synonyms. Phthisis of the larynx. Consumption of the throat.

Etiology. Nearly all cases of tuberculosis of the larynx show a predisposition to catarrhal conditions of the mucous membrane of the throat. Inherited delicacy and all acquired conditions and occupations that predispose to lowered physical vitality are to be considered as etiological factors.

In primary tuberculosis the tubercle-bacilli undoubtedly gain entrance from without. But in the large majority of cases, laryngeal tuberculosis is a secondary manifestation of the same disease in other organs, usually the lungs.

Symptoms. In many cases the onset of the disease is insidious. The voice easily tires on exertion, the cough is of a paroxysmal character with little or no expectoration. Unilateral smarting or burning is frequent. In suspected cases, pronounced irritation on one side of the throat should always lead to a thorough examination, as this symptom is strongly suspicious of incipient laryngeal tuberculosis.

As the disease progresses, the cough and pain on swallowing increase. The latter condition may become intense when the epiglottis is ulcerated. When the pharyngo-epiglottic folds and border of the epiglottis are ulcerated, the pain extends to the ear on the affected side. Not infrequently the uvula becomes decidedly club-shaped. The swelling of the soft tissues may prevent complete closure of the glottis, so that efforts in swallowing liquids may cause severe attacks of coughing. Expectoration may not be free until ulceration is extensive, or until the lungs are greatly involved. During the early stage increased pulse and a slight rise in temperature are present. Gradually there supervenes emaciation, great prostration, hectic, etc.

Examination with the laryngoscope reveals the epiglottis thickened and assuming a thick roll, the so-called turban or horse-shoe shape. The ary-epiglottic folds become enlarged. When the cartilages of Santorini and Wrisberg are involved in the œdematous swelling, the disease is assuredly tuberculosis.

During the later stages of prolonged cases, chondritis and perichondritis are frequent complications; fragments of the necrosed cartilage are sometimes seen projecting into the larynx.

Diagnosis. The disease with which laryngeal phthisis is most apt to be confronted is syphilis. The differential diagnosis is not always as readily made as some authors claim. The two diseases present many symptoms in common. One condition I have invariably noticed in tuberculosis is, a prominence in the throat of the cervical vertebræ.

The following, modified from Bosworth, may assist in the diagnosis. In phthisis the ulcer has irregular edges, is not deeply excavated, there is not a clear line of demarcation, and the mucus is grayish, ropy in character. The ulcer extends slowly and is superficial. The aid furnished by the microscope is invaluable.

The syphilitic ulcer has sharp-cut edges and is deeply excavated; is rapidly destructive; the areola is deep red angry-looking, and the line of demarcation is usually distinct. The secretion is yellow, purulent. Other symptoms of syphilis can be obtained. Syphilis, as a rule, quickly responds to proper treatment, the improvement not infrequently taking place within four days.

Prognosis. The prognosis is usually grave, but not necessarily fatal. During the last few years local treatment, conjoined with internal medicine, has cured many cases, and in the vast majority of instances has served to prolong life and alleviate the intense suffering so characteristic of the disease.

In those rare cases where syphilis and tuberculosis co-exist, the result is fatal.

Treatment, The general treatment, in the main, is the same as the treatment employed in pulmonary tuberculosis. One additional point is to be emphasized, namely, the voice must be kept at rest.

Over-bundling the neck and too close confinement within doors are to be avoided.

Constant coddling tends to make invalids of persons who are well, and to increase invalidism in those who are already sick. Unless the condition is making rapid progress an outdoor life is sometimes advisable. Other things being equal, the patient, if a man, will, in many instances, do far better by roughing it in the pine woods of our Northern States. At least such a life can take the consumptive off no quicker than living in overheated rooms, as he is prone to do when at home.

In cases in which the pulmonary disease is not active, the method practiced by Hering and Krause of curetting the diseased tissue, and then applying lactic acid, has proven of decided benefit. The curetting and applications are to be made with specially devised instruments. Cocaine anæsthesia is necessary. The diseased tissue must be removed, first attacking the parts interfering with respiration. The denuded surface is then thoroughly rubbed with lactic acid, beginning with a twenty per cent. and gradually increasing to a seventy per cent. solution. To avoid infection of the wound, as soon as bleeding has ceased, it is to be painted with a one to two per cent. solution of pyoktanin. If an inflammatory irritation ensues the pyoktanin solution has been too strong. The scraped surface frequently heals in from one to two weeks. I am certain that this is a valuable method of treating laryngeal tuberculosis, but I desire to emphasize the fact that to be successful it must be thoroughly understood, and that it can be successfully applied only by the physician who is familiar with making local applications to the throat.

Other methods will sometimes afford relief, as daily injection into the larynx of a twenty per cent. menthol in albolene. When the surface is unbroken, favorable results have been claimed from daily application of creosote five minims, iodine five grains, and iodide of potash twenty grains, to glycerine one ounce.

When ulceration has taken place, insufflations of one of the various iodine preparations on the market, or swabbing the surface with iodoform one part to sulphuric ether fifteen parts, may be used. Competent observers have frequently reported favorable results following the internal and topical use of creosote.

If dysphagia is extreme, morphia one to four grains to the ounce of water; or cocaine in the same strength, may be applied by atomizer, or applicator, ten to fifteen minutes before eating, or as is necessary.

Codeine, one-fourth grain, will often assist in controlling the dry, tickling cough at night. Remedies of this character should be used only as a last resort.

Hypodermic injection as advocated by Koch has not maintained its position as a curative agent that its early supporters hoped for, yet favorable reports from its use are, from time to time, reported in the medical journals. It is my opinion, based on personal experience, that better results are obtained from *Bacillinum* in a medium to a high potency.

Therapeutics

Arsenicum iod. Arytenoids anæmic and puffy; œdematous condition of mucous membrane; chondritis and perichondritis; sero-purulent secretion; voice weak and trembling. Emaciation and prostration marked.

Drosera. Constriction of larynx when talking; sensation of a feather in the throat, exciting cough; voice hoarse, deep; great exertion to speak. Talking aggravates the throat symptoms.

Iodium. Tightness and constriction about larynx with hoarseness, may be complete aphonia; ulceration, with abundant secretion; constant hemming and hawking.

Silicea. Ulceration of the cartilages; hoarseness, roughness and dryness in the throat, with irritating cough; or, cough may be racking and loose with copious expectoration of thick, yellow pus, accompanied with hectic night sweats and great debility.

Stannum. Constant, short, irritating, hacking cough and aphonia, with empty feeling in the chest.

Consult *Bacillinum, Calcarea carb., Calcarea phos., Phosphorus, Psorinum* and *Sanguinaria.*

Chapter XIX

TUMORS OF THE LARYNX

(benign tumors)

Papillomata or *warty growths* are the most common. This form of tumor shows a preference for young adults. The tumors are usually sessile, varying in size from the head of a pin to a mass filling the glottis. Their color is generally pale pink, and they present a warty or cauliflower-like surface.

Their usual point of attachment is the free border of the vocal cords. As they frequently return after removal they should be closely watched, and on their reappearance should again be removed.

Treatment. The instruments necessary for their removal are snares, forceps and specially devised knives.

Therapeutics

Compare *Thuja*, *Causticum*, *Kali bich.*, and *Sanguinaria*.

Fibromata are of a pinkish color and are firmer to pressure than papilloma, though somewhat resembling the latter in appearance. Fibromata are sometimes pedunculated, or their point of attachment may be only slightly constricted; they are usually attached to one of the vocal cords. They rarely recur after removal.

Treatment. This consists in removal by snare or forceps.

Cystoma is the result of occlusion of a muciparous gland on the epiglottis, or ventricular bands. The tumor is globular in form with a smooth surface.

The treatment consists in opening the cyst by means of a guarded knife. After escape of its contents the inner wall of the sac should be painted with iodine.

MALIGNANT TUMORS

Carcinoma of the larynx invariably occurs after the fortieth year of age.

Epithelioma and *Encephaloid*. These forms of cancer are the most common. Their usual seat of growth is on the vocal cords, the epiglottis, or on the ventricular bands. But in many cases the surrounding tissues quickly become infiltrated so that the primary seat of the disease cannot always be determined. When the epiglottis is attacked it may become so swollen as to prevent a view of the larynx.

Symptoms. In many cases there will be a history of slight hoarseness existing for months, or years before the appearance of the disease. Later the hoarseness increases, although the voice is rarely entirely lost. Dyspnœa increases as the tumor encroaches on the glottic orifice. When ulceration begins, pain of a lancinating character is common, although not always present. As the disease advances, expectoration becomes fetid, purulent and occasionally mixed with blood. Increased flow of saliva is always present. When the epiglottis and the arytenoid region are involved, painful deglutition is an early symptom.

Cancer presents a grayish-white or deeply-red color, with a ragged, uneven surface.

Sarcoma. This form of tumor in the larynx is very rare. The vocal cords are seldom attacked. The tumor is smooth and somewhat globular in form.

Diagnosis of Malignant Tumors. In the early stage the differential diagnosis is often difficult.' Malignant disease may be mistaken for syphilis, and tuberculosis.

The microscope will assist in differentiating benign growths. When the diagnosis is uncertain, anti-syphilitic treatment should be tried.

Prognosis. Epithelioma, and encephaloid cancer are invariably fatal. Where sarcoma has invaded the surounding tissue the result is fatal. But where the tumor is unilateral, and there is slight infiltration, thorough removal holds out some hope of relief.

Treatment. Surgical treatment should be undertaken only during the early manifestations of the disease. Endo-laryngeal operations, either by cutting or by the galvano-cautery, have given the best results.

Extirpation of the larynx has given relief in a very few cases, but the majority of patients quickly succumb as the result of the operation.

A low tracheotomy is frequently demanded for the relief of respiratory obstruction. Life may be prolonged several months as a result of the artificial opening.

For further treatment and therapeutics consult Malignant Tumors of the Nose.

Chapter XX

NEUROSES OF THE LARYNX

(PARALYSIS)

Paralysis of Adduction is due to a paralysis of the lateral crico-arytenoid muscles.

Etiology. This condition may be caused by catarrhal inflammation, anæmia, rheumatism, hysteria, and over-exertion of the voice, as in shouting. Lead or arsenic poisoning may cause it.

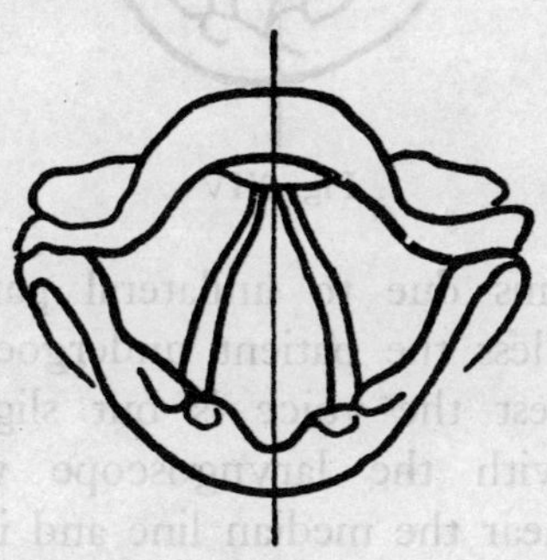

Fig. XIII

Symptoms. If bilateral paralysis exists the cords will be seen widely separated, and the voice is entirely lost. The effort to whisper or cough causes great fatigue.

Prognosis. Usually favorable.

Paralysis of Abduction is due to paralysis of the posterior crico-arytenoid muscles.

Etiology. This form of paralysis rarely involves both sides of the larynx. It is usually unilateral, and may be due to some lesion of the pneumogastric; to aneurism of the carotid artery; or to carcinoma of the œsophagus. It may be the result of pressure from an enlarged thyroid gland. In children enlarged bronchial, and cervical glands may be the cause. A few cases have followed typhoid fever.

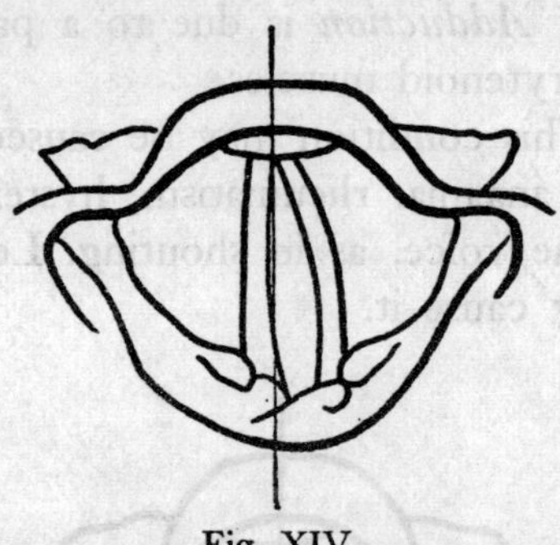

Fig. XIV

The symptoms due to unilateral paralysis are not pronounced unless the patient undergoes violent exercise. During rest the voice is but slightly impaired. Examination with the laryngoscope will show the affected cord near the median line and immovable.

In bilateral paralysis both cords are fixed in the median line, and are separated by a very narrow space.

Prognosis. Both conditions, but especially the bilateral form of the disease, are exceedingly grave. Tracheotomy may be suddenly demanded to prevent suffocation.

Paralysis of the crico-thyroid is exceedingly rare.

Paralysis of the thyro-arytenoids is not uncommon.

Etiology. This condition is usually caused by chronic inflammation of the larynx. Or it may be due to straining, or excessive use of the voice.

Symptoms. The voice is husky and weak. When bilateral an elliptical space can be seen separating the cords during phonation.

Prognosis. The result is usually favorable, but in chronic cases the hoarseness may be permanent.

Total paralysis of one vocal cord, or *laryngo-hemiplegia*. Ordinary conversation is sometimes possible, but decided hoarseness is usual, and the voice easily tires when used.

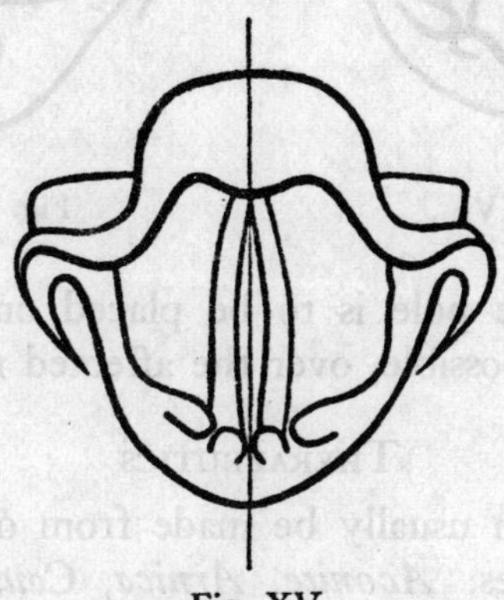

Fig. XV

Prognosis. Relief will usually be obtained within three or four months, or not at all.

Treatment. The treatment necessarily depends on the cause; this should be sought for in all cases.

Stimulation of the muscles by the electrical current is often advisable. When applying electricity to the larynx, weak current should always be used for the first few treatments, and each treatment no longer than four or five seconds.

The negative electrode may be placed on the posterior laryngeal wall; the positive pole placed on the neck over the course of the recurrent nerve. In some cases benefit will follow the external application of the

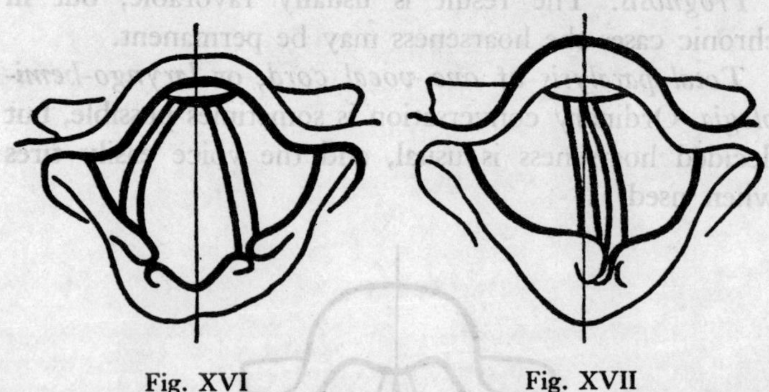

Fig. XVI Fig. XVII

electrodes. One pole is to be placed on each side of the larynx, if possible, over the affected muscle.

Therapeutics

A choice can usually be made from one of the following remedies: *Aconite*, *Arnica*, *Causticum*, *Gelsemium*, *Ignatia*, *Oxalic acid*, *Rhus tox.*, *Selenium*, and *Senega*.

HYPERÆSTHESIA

Oversensitiveness of the mucous membrane of the larynx, is present in inflammatory conditions, and ulcerations. Or, it may be symptomatic of hysteria.

ANÆSTHESIA

Loss of sensation may be limited to a small portion of the larynx, as the epiglottis, or the supra-glottic region; or, it may be complete, involving the whole of the larynx.

The causes are chronic inflammations, trauma, diphtheria, and syphilis. Or, it may be central in origin.

PARÆSTHESIA

Perverted or abnormal sensations in the larynx are rarely accompanied by pain.

The sensation may be due to a foreign body irritating the larynx, which is subsequently expelled or swallowed.

Localized inflammations, especially enlarged glands, or follicles, are often causes of peculiar sensations in the throat. Many cases are reflex from flatulence in the stomach or bowels. Irritation of the rectum may likewise produce it. Or, the sensation may be wholly neurotic in origin. In women the sensory neuroses are frequently aggravated during the menstrual period.

Treatment. In all cases the causes should be ascertained, and appropriate treatment directed toward its removal. When symptoms of a neurotic character are present, the potentized remedy will frequently prove sufficient.

THERAPEUTICS

Consult *Aconite*, *Asafœtida*, *Gelsemium*, *Ignatia*. *Moschus*, *Platina* and *Sepia*.

INDEX